SOMATIC THERAPY FOR TRAUMA

| A 28-DAY PROGRAM |
FROM CHAOS TO CONNECTION |
NERVOUS SYSTEM REGULATION
WITH SOMATIC EXPERIENCING EXERCISES

ADELE WILSON

MY ZEN POWER TRIBE PUBLISHING

ISBN Number 9798326246783

DISCLAIMER/Legal Notice

The information provided in this book is for educational and informational purposes only.

It is not intended to be a substitute for professional medical advice, diagnosis, or treatment. Always seek the advice of your physician or other qualified health provider with questions you may have regarding a medical condition.

The author and publisher of this book are not responsible for any adverse effects or consequences resulting from the use of the information provided in this book. The reader assumes full responsibility for their actions and decisions based on the content of this book.

If you are experiencing a medical or mental health emergency, please seek immediate assistance from a qualified healthcare professional or contact your local emergency services.

"When things change inside you, things change around you."

—Unknown

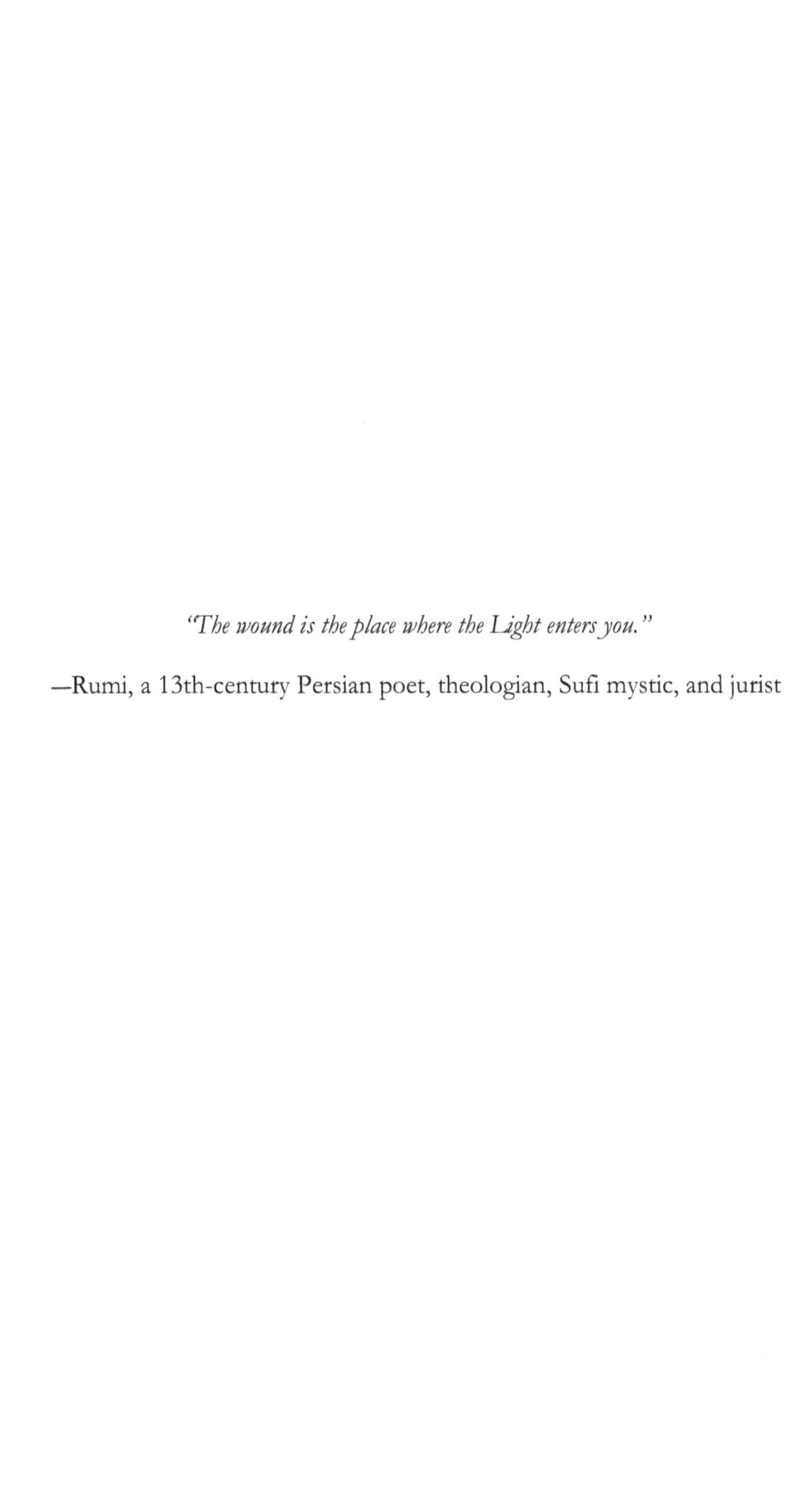

"The wound is the place where the Light enters you."

—Rumi, a 13th-century Persian poet, theologian, Sufi mystic, and jurist

"You are not alone. You are not crazy.
There is a rational explanation for what is happening to you.
You have not been irreversibly damaged,
and it is possible to diminish or even eliminate your symptoms."

—Peter A. Levine, Ph. D. from *Waking The Tiger*

I dedicate this book to *you*, my dear.

It takes courage to start the journey towards healing, because often it requires us to step outside the normal, the boring, the lovely little setup called everyday life.

It takes courage to decide to heal.

You have taken the first step. You are truly a real-life superhero.

I would also like to dedicate this book to all you beautiful, courageous clients. I treat your trust with my deepest, heartfelt gratefulness.

Also, I dedicate this book to my lovely family, who have beared with me on my worst, celebrated with me on my best, and with whom I am blessed to share this beautiful hike called life.

Thank you, B.

BUT FIRST: YOUR FREE GIFT

Firstly, my dear, we want you to have a free gift as a thank you for stepping in.

We believe healing and creating our dream lives are actually very close to one another, since dreams (or goals, if you will) fuel the healing and vice versa. Looking to the future is as important as looking at and healing from our past.

Sometimes we need to heal first to really find our dream life, and sometimes we need dreams to support our healing.

Our free gift for you helps you with creating your dream life.

Sign in our website www.myzenpower.co

And you will get a FREE eBook: Step-by-Step Guide to Create Your Dream Life!

But there is more! You will also get sneak peaks, free copies of our future books, and healing information... Plus a loving tribe of like-minded friends on the same journey. Welcome, my dear.

We hope this journey we share is only the first journey together. We believe in creating our dream lives, and it can happen through healing and, for example, envisioning our dream life—we believe we all are worth finding the magic in our lives.

INTRODUCTION: WHO WE ARE

We at My Zen Power Tribe Publishing believe in healing and that it can come in so many beautiful forms. The reason there are so many methods is that we humans come in so many plentiful forms. To us, we are happy with any kind of healing, coming from any method, therapist, or author, as long as it's truly healing for our reader. We thank all you therapists, healers, and authors out there for sharing the same passion.

We believe in healing, supporting us in creating our dream lives. We believe we all deserve to live the fullest, happiest, and most fulfilling lives. Sometimes life invites us to work with our underlying traumas before we are able to feel worthy to receive the life we have always wanted.

WHAT THEY SAY ABOUT US

As a quite fresh publisher, you might wonder what people say about us. We have been fortunate to have beautiful feedback, which we are deeply grateful for. Your words give our work a deeper meaning, giving us so much courage in those days when we have doubts like we all do sometimes: *Why do I do this? Does anyone care? Does this make any difference of any kind?*

FIVE STARS

"This book can seriously be life-changing! You share so many amazing tools to help readers have a better life!"
—Susan K, about this book

"...this guidebook provides a clear pathway from the outset. It's very informative while still being accessible, taking the time to explain the principles of shadow work, how it works, and why it's used."...

"I especially appreciated the more light-hearted and casual tone of the writing throughout.

You can find more information about your publisher at the end of this book.

YOUR AUTHOR

Adele Wilson has worked as a counselor for well over a two decades and holds a degree in psychology. She is specialized in somatic experiencing and creative healing methods especially in trauma healing. Her deepest passion is to help others. She also is an experienced meditator as well as a yoga and *pranayama* instructor. In her work, she aims to help people to reconnect their minds and bodies with compassion and love, and with trauma awareness as the working method to heal traumas. Adele is also an author, a mother of three beautiful kids, and in her free time, a passionate dog trainer.

She also is a fellow trauma survivor, so she knows both the professional and the emotional sides of trauma healing, and with this book wanted to give you the tools she has professionally and personally found the most effective.

She loves her work, and she believes in the support of women supporting women. She deeply believes in Zen Power Tribe's rule:

"A glowing woman can help other women glow and still be lit."

— Unknown (Fellow Hero!)

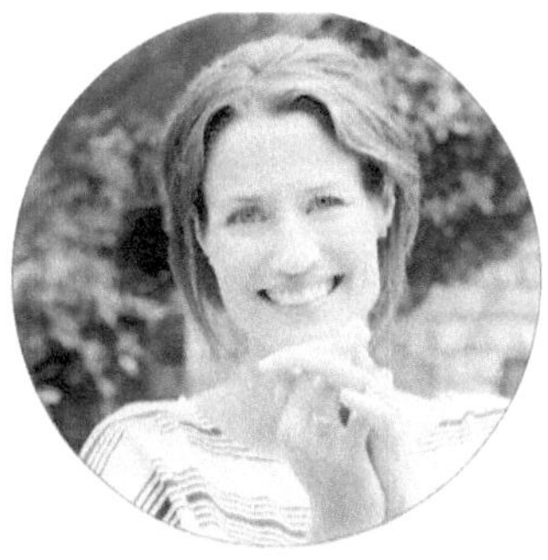

FOREWORD ONE

Someone very wise has said: There is only two places you need to go often. The place what heals you, and the place what inspires you.

This book, from my view, is both of those places.

It is (indeed!) with great honor to write this foreword for Adele Wilson's beautiful book on somatic therapy. As a yoga instructor and fellow author, I have had the privilege of witnessing Adele's profound journey of healing and transformation, both as a counselor–and most importantly, as a fellow trauma survivor.

I believe it takes one to know one.

What, from my view, sets Adele apart is their ability to create a beautiful, safe, and nurturing space for you to heal. Her compassionate approach invites you to explore your own story with kindness and without judgment, creating an environment where true healing can happen. This book is not just a manual; it is a companion on your journey, what offers support and love every step of the way.

Healing is not a destination but a journey, one that is best undertaken with the support of a compassionate guide. Adele's work embodies this philosophy, reminding us of one of the most important things in trauma healing: we are never alone on our path.

I loved this book. I loved the hope, the compassion, the humor. I loved the feeling I was not alone.

I hope you will too.

With love,

Claudia Berg

Fellow Author, Yoga Instructor

FOREWORD TWO

Being invited to write the foreword for this book has been an honor, as I get to help others see the magic of somatic healing. I am a licensed mental health therapist who works with individuals who have experienced trauma, and I am very excited to have accessible resources, such as this workbook, for those who want to find relief.

By utilizing this book, you are choosing to reclaim your power and connect with the essence of who you are while leaving the hurt behind you.

I've seen just how often trauma can feel like it has a crippling hold on you and your life. I am so happy to know this book is designed to help you wiggle free from the pain, let go, and feel more like yourself. Psychological impacts of trauma can be detrimental, and equally as important is how the body responds and reacts to traumatic experiences. Many therapists, including myself, incorporate the use of somatic exercises into their practice with clients. Somatic work is one of the top interventions that professionals use while treating trauma-related symptoms in people with post-traumatic disorders. These exercises are designed to help you create more awareness in your body, allowing you to further gain insight into your emotions and thought processes. Once the awareness is created, you will learn how to accept, regulate, and even release the trauma that your body has stored. Similar to a therapy session, this book will guide through various methods of somatic healing. I tend to share with many of my clients that healing the mind also comes from healing the body.

Experiences of adverse events lead the human body to flip into fight, flight or freeze mode, also known as survival mode. Oftentimes people have been living in survival mode for a very long time. When this happens, the sympathetic nervous system is activated. This is the mechanism in the human body that increases heart rate, raises blood pressure, creates more blood flow to muscles, and leaves us feeling on edge, fidgety, and unable to relax. Using the assessment tools, questionnaires, exercises, and other resources in this book, you will learn to regulate the sympathetic nervous system and activate your parasympathetic nervous system, or the mechanism that promotes relaxation, restoration, and calmness. Mental health professionals like myself tend to make grounding a foundation of our work with clients.

We are so happy you are choosing to live life on your terms and using this guide in your healing journey. As you reflect, process, grow and heal, we want to remind you to check in with your body often throughout the day. This promotes healthy regulation and more opportunities to ground yourself in the present moment. I'd invite you to offer yourself grace in this journey of rebirth, as you are human, and you are working through a process. Finding peace amongst one or multiple traumatic events looks different for all, so it is okay to be gentle with yourself during this time.

Alyssa Biestek

Licensed marriage and family therapist (LMFT)

TABLE OF CONTENTS

AUTHOR'S NOTE:

WHY I WROTE THIS BOOK

Welcome, my dear.

I am so glad you are here. You have taken the first step towards healing—the kindness, happiness, and joy.

The first step is always the most important! Many people don't have the courage to take the first step. So, in my opinion, you can already celebrate yourself as a superhero.

But it gets better. I hope this book serves you and keeps you good company on your journey towards *your* healing and better life. (*Yours*, and no one else's!)

We wanted to create not just a somatic therapy book, but a loving guide. A guide, a companion, sometimes asking persistent or even weird questions, but always with one purpose: supporting you on your healing journey, always with love. Please, my dear, remember: You have the inner knowing in you. Move at your own pace. There is absolutely no rush. Even though I built this as a 30-day journey, there is absolutely no problem if you want to change the pace. You know best what is best for you.

The reason I wrote this book is very simple. I have worked with clients for over two decades, and I have always thought about what I could do more. I wanted to give back, since I feel I have had so much help over the years: from colleagues, from those clearing the path in front of me, researchers, clients, fellow humans. I am deeply thankful for all my friends, scientists, therapists, trainers, and fellow travelers who have guided me in the right direction, given me ideas, empowering me when I was down, and celebrating with me on the high notes. Thank you.

That direction has led me to study the human mind and body and how to help them to get connected and by doing that, helping to heal. Together.

I wrote this book in a common language, on purpose, since I would be delighted to serve as many of you as possible: adults, parents, children, teachers, people working with children. (We have a somatic therapy book for children coming, but in the meantime, you may alter some of the exercises in this book also for kids.)

This book is an overview of somatic therapy, and my goal is to help you find an easy way to get your healing journey started.

Each one of the topics in this book deserves a chapter or even a book of their own. Please understand, each one of the topics is huge and important, including so much potential to heal—but also, we need to remember I wanted to give you an overview and necessary and powerful tools to start your healing journey, so I needed to keep each topic in an easy digestible form.

I decided to build a simple, quick, but deeply powerful 30-day somatic therapy program for you to start your healing journey. I will give you simple exercises to step on your path, and my deepest hope is that this book can help you find your joy and your own path, and the empowerment to carry on. (We also will have other books for you to continue with us, if you feel this path is inviting.)

I wanted to give you a comprehensive, loving overview, an easily digestible 30-day somatic therapy program, complete with experiencing exercises. I wanted engaging in this program to be easy to adapt to your daily life. Each day's exercises are planned to be easily practiced. If you are very busy, you'll be able to do your day's exercises even in 10 to 15 minutes. On top of this, I wanted to give you deeper knowledge and more exercises, if you want.

Trust your inner wisdom. As Peter A. Levine so beautifully words it: Trauma does not have to be a life-sentence. Instead, it can guide us to a beautiful transformation.

I wish you the most wonderful outcomes. Remember, you're not alone on this journey. We're here with you, cheering you on, and celebrating every moment of your healing. You rock!

So, welcome, my dear. Please feel free to take what you feel useful and leave the rest.

With love,

Adele

Author, Counselor, Fellow Traveler

My Zen Power Tribe Publishing

PART I

TEST: COULD SOMATIC THERAPY BE A FIT FOR YOU?

You might be like most of us: trying to enter and walk on our healing journey, but drowning in all the information, instructions, ideas, thoughts, and advice. Advice floods us from social media gurus, algorithms, and all the junk we face in our daily lives. Unless, of course, you live in the Himalayas as a monk, but most of us don't.

I have good news for you: For healing, my dear, you don't have to live in the Himalayas. You can heal from past traumas and all the junk in so many ways, which one might be somatic therapy. You are welcomed to take this test and see if this healing method would be a good fit for you.

This test is a quick one. It only takes a few minutes to complete.

TEST INSTRUCTIONS

1. Please set aside a quiet, uninterrupted, and peaceful time to complete the test.

2. Read each question carefully and answer honestly based on your own experiences and feelings.

3. Choose the response that best reflects your thoughts or behaviors.

4. Once you've completed all the questions, tally your "yes" responses.

5. Refer to the scoring guide to interpret your results and determine whether somatic therapy may align with your needs and interests.

6. Remember, this quiz is simply a tool to help you gain insight into whether somatic therapy could be a beneficial addition to your healing journey. Trust yourself, honor your truth, and know that support and guidance are available whenever you're ready to take the next step.

1. **Do you experience physical symptoms of stress or trauma, such as tension, headaches, or digestive issues?**

    - Yes

    - No

2. **Are you interested in exploring the connection between your emotions and physical sensations?**

    - Yes

    - No

3. **Do you feel disconnected from your body or struggle to regulate your emotions?**

    - Yes

    - No

4. **Have you experienced trauma or adverse life events that continue to affect you emotionally and physically?**

    - Yes

    - No

5. **Are you open to trying holistic approaches to mental health that incorporate the body's wisdom?**

   - Yes

   - No

6. **Do you prefer therapy techniques that involve both verbal communication and body-centered approaches?**

   - Yes

   - No

7. **Are you seeking relief from chronic pain, anxiety, or depression?**

   - Yes

   - No

8. **Would you be willing to engage in exercises or practices that focus on bodily sensations and movement?**

   - Yes

   - No

9. **Do you believe that past experiences can manifest in physical symptoms and affect your wellbeing?**

   - Yes

   - No

10. **Are you committed to the process of self-discovery and personal growth?**

    - Yes

    - No

SCORING THE TEST

- Count the number of "yes" responses. How many did you get? Write it down, if you wish.

- If you answered "yes" to fewer than six questions, somatic therapy might not align with your preferences and needs.

- If you answered "yes" to six or more questions, somatic therapy may be a good fit for you.

- Or, simply, if you feel somatic therapy might be something you want to try, don't mind the amount of yesses or no's, just simply step in. Trust your inner guidance, my dear!

Somatic therapy focuses on the mind-body connection and may offer valuable tools for individuals seeking holistic approaches to mental health and wellbeing. Thank you for taking the time to explore whether somatic therapy may be a good fit for you. Remember, the journey towards healing and self-discovery is a deeply personal one, and it's important to find approaches that resonate with your unique needs and preferences.

TEST CONCLUSION

As you reflect on your responses to the test, you might want to consider the following thoughts:

- Embrace the power of the mind-body connection: Somatic therapy offers a holistic approach to healing, acknowledging the interplay between our physical sensations and emotional wellbeing.

- Trust your intuition: If you feel drawn to explore somatic therapy further, trust that inner knowing. Our intuition often guides us towards what we truly need.

- Cultivate self-compassion: Regardless of your test results, remember to be gentle with yourself. Healing is a journey, and every single step you take towards greater self-awareness and self-care is a triumph to celebrate. You, my dear, are a REAL super hero!

Q&A OF SOMATIC THERAPY

There are so many therapy methods (and so many questions about each one of them!), and we wanted you to have a quick overview of somatic therapy. We didn't want to send you on just by yourself: we wanted to share some of the common questions and answers that might help you and/or provide an answer for a question even you might not have asked.

1. **What is somatic therapy?**

   My dear, somatic therapy is a holistic approach to healing that focuses on the mind-body connection, addressing psychological issues through bodily sensations and movements. So, somatic therapy, from my perspective, respects the fact that we are a whole being, instead of a carry bag for our brain, or vice versa.

2. **What benefits can I expect from a 30-day somatic therapy program?**

   My dear, so many! After completing a 30-day somatic therapy program, you may experience several benefits, such as:

3. **Reduced Stress and Anxiety**

   Somatic therapy helps regulate the nervous system, leading to decreased stress and anxiety levels.

Improved Emotional Regulation

Through somatic techniques, you'll learn to identify and manage emotions effectively, promoting emotional balance.

4. **Enhanced Mind-Body Connection**
   Somatic therapy fosters a deeper understanding of the connection between physical sensations and emotions, leading to improved self-awareness.

5. **Trauma Resolution**
   If you've experienced trauma, somatic therapy can aid in processing and releasing trauma from the body, facilitating healing.

6. **Better Physical Health**
   By addressing physical manifestations of stress and trauma, such as muscle tension, somatic therapy can contribute to overall physical wellbeing.

7. **Increased Resilience**
   Building resilience is a key outcome of somatic therapy, empowering you to cope with life's challenges more effectively.

In conclusion, embarking on a 30-day somatic therapy program can lead to significant improvements in both mental and physical wellbeing, providing you with the gorgeous invaluable tools to navigate life with greater ease and resilience. Sounds pretty good to me. What do you think?

1. **And how does it work then? Somatic therapy, I mean?**
   Somatic therapy works by exploring bodily sensations and

experiences to release tension, regulate emotions, and promote overall wellbeing.

2. What issues can somatic therapy help with?

Somatic therapy can help with a wide range of issues, including trauma, stress, anxiety, depression, chronic pain, and emotional regulation.

3. What techniques can be used in somatic therapy?

Techniques used in somatic therapy many times include mindfulness, breathwork, body awareness exercises, movement therapy, and touch therapy.

4. Is somatic therapy suitable for everyone?

Somatic therapy can benefit people of all ages and backgrounds. But, as always, it's good to bear in mind, it may not be suitable for everyone. It's always useful, and in some cases, essential to consult with a qualified therapist to determine suitability. I cannot emphasize enough, we are all individuals, and the same methods might have a different effect on us—so, please my dear, listen to yourself and respect your inner wisdom.

5. How long does somatic therapy take to see results?

The duration of somatic therapy varies depending on the individual and the issues being addressed. Some people may see results in a few sessions, while others may require longer-term therapy.

6. Is somatic therapy painful?

Somatic therapy should absolutely not be painful. It focuses on creating a safe and supportive environment for healing, and therapists prioritize the client's comfort and wellbeing.

7. What should I expect in a somatic therapy session?

In a somatic therapy session, you can expect to explore bodily sensations, movements, and experiences guided by a trained therapist. Sessions may include verbal dialogue, mindfulness exercises, and physical interventions.

8. Can somatic therapy be done online?

Yes, somatic therapy can, many times, be conducted online through, for example, video conferencing platforms. However, some physical techniques may be adapted or modified for online sessions. And we always have to remember, person to person is almost always better, safer, more efficient and... more human. But as we may not always have the luxury of choice, online therapies might work as well, especially as a supportive form.

9. How do I find a qualified somatic therapist?

To find a qualified somatic therapist, you can ask for recommendations from healthcare professionals, search online directories, or contact professional associations for referrals. Personally, I suggest contacting professional associations or healthcare professionals, or check online therapy candidates' track records.

10. Is somatic therapy covered by insurance?

Coverage for somatic therapy varies depending on your insurance provider and policy. I'd say it's advisable to check with your insurance company to determine coverage options.

11. Are there any side effects of somatic therapy?

Side effects of somatic therapy are generally considered to be mild and/or temporary. They may include heightened emotions, physical discomfort, or fatigue, but these usually subside with time. Please, if at any point you experience unbearable discomfort, please seek professional support, as there are highly skillful therapists trained to help and support.

12. How does somatic therapy differ from traditional talk therapy?

Somatic therapy differs from traditional talk therapy by incorporating the body's experiences and sensations into the therapeutic process, whereas talk therapy primarily focuses on verbal dialogue. There are pros and cons to each, and I would again say to trust the inner guidance.

13. Can somatic therapy help with trauma recovery?

Yes, somatic therapy is considered being highly effective for trauma recovery. It helps with processing traumatic experiences stored in the body, releases trauma-related tension, and restores a sense of safety and empowerment. I personally have my own professional experience of this on both sides of the glass, and I have experienced the incredible healing powers of its holistic approach.

14. Is somatic therapy evidence-based?

Yes, somatic therapy has a growing body of research supporting its effectiveness in treating various mental health conditions, including trauma, anxiety, and depression. If you are interested in this particular topic, you can find more information, for example *Harvard Health Publication* and *Forbes* (the links are in the references).

15. What qualifications do somatic therapists have?

Somatic therapists typically have training in psychology, counseling, or body-centered modalities such as Somatic Experiencing, Sensorimotor Psychotherapy, or Hakomi Therapy.

16. Can somatic therapy be integrated with other forms of therapy?

Yes, somatic therapy can be integrated with other forms of therapy, such as cognitive-behavioral therapy (CBT), mindfulness-based therapies, and expressive arts therapy to enhance treatment outcomes. In my opinion, somatic therapy is easily connected to other healing therapies.

17. Is somatic therapy suitable for children?

Yes, somatic therapy can be beneficial for children, especially those who have experienced trauma or have difficulty expressing their emotions verbally. I would advise paying extra attention when choosing the right therapy method for a child, since childhood is such a delicate time.

18. What role does the therapist play in somatic therapy?

The therapist in somatic therapy serves simply as a guide and facilitator, creating a safe and supportive environment for clients to explore their bodily experiences and emotions.

19. **How can I learn more about somatic therapy?**

You can learn more about somatic therapy by researching online resources*, reading books on the topic, attending workshops or seminars, and consulting with qualified somatic therapists. *You know this, but I can't stress it enough: please have some healthy criticism with online sources, since all are not dependable. (While some fortunately are!)

SELF-ASSESSMENT SCORING BEFORE (AND AFTER) YOUR SOMATIC JOURNEY

Somatic therapy recognizes the profound connection between our physical sensations, emotions, and overall wellbeing.

Self-assessment can be an important component of our somatic therapy journey by inviting us to explore our internal experiences before and after our journey. It can help us see the self-discovery, growth, and healing—the transformation! —we have gained through our heroic path. You can look at it as a compass that can guide you towards greater insight into your life and healing.

Self-assessment can provide us with an opportunity to lovingly observe ourselves. By acknowledging and honoring our experiences, we can release stored tension, rewire neural pathways, and foster a sense of wholeness and integration. Through self-assessment, we can witness our sometimes-profound transformation and inner peace during our somatic therapy exercises journey.

These 10 self-assessment questions can guide you to evaluate your situation before and after our journey.

1. On a scale of 1-10, how would you rate your overall level of physical tension or discomfort?

2. How intense are your bodily sensations when experiencing stress or anxiety? Rate from 1 to 10.

3. To what extent do you feel connected to your body on a daily basis? Rate from 1 (not at all) to 10 (very connected).

4. How would you rate your awareness of bodily sensations, such as muscle tension or heart rate changes? Use a scale of 1-10.

5. On a scale of 1-10, how present are you in your body during moments of emotional distress?

6. How comfortable do you feel expressing emotions physically (e.g., through gestures or body movements)? Rate from 1 to 10.

7. To what extent do you notice changes in your breathing patterns during times of stress? Rate from 1 (not noticeable) to 10 (highly noticeable).

8. How frequently do you experience physical symptoms, such as headaches or stomachaches, related to stress or emotional triggers? Rate from 1 to 10.

9. On a scale of 1-10, how often do you notice feelings of joy and peace?

10. To what extent do you feel grounded and present in your body? Use a scale of 1-10.

Just for you to have an idea of your journey and how it has affected you, we will ask these questions again at the end of the book. Sometimes, seeing where we came from and where we are now can be truly transformational.

PART II

"The mind and body are a powerful duo. Keep them in harmony."
—Unknown

WHAT YOU WILL GET WITH THIS BOOK

Thank you for coming in. You really are a superhero! The journey we are about to start together can be partly challenging, but I hope at the end you'll find it was worth every moment.

So, in brief, with this book, you will get:

- 30-day somatic therapy program.
- 10-15 minutes somatic experiencing exercises each day.
- Extra information and exercises.
- Bonuses.
- Understanding and guidance about somatic therapy.
- Instructions on how to do the exercises.
- Tools, tools, tools.
- Self-assessment tools for you to see how your journey has affected you.
- Gentle guidance starting with easier exercises and deepening them.
- **Loving cheering** on the way. **(All somatic therapy doers are heroes.)**

Understanding and support to get through your 30-day somatic therapy journey and **get to the other side**—to the self-love, joy, and happiness.

With this book, you will understand:

- **What somatic therapy is** and where it originated from—and how it looks in its simplest form.
- **How our past traumas affect our behavior.** (Even if we might try to ignore them; at least I have, but they are persistent and won't just go away.)
- Is somatic therapy **suitable** for you?
- **Benefits of somatic therapy.**
- The **key elements and mindset** in successful somatic therapy.
- **How to** do somatic therapy (we guide you). Q&A's!
- **Integrating** your new self into your life with self-love!

THE POWER OF INTENTION SETTING IN SOMATIC THERAPY

Our intention is behind every action we take. Every single one! It can be conscious or unconscious, but it's there. And yet it can often be one of the most underestimated areas of our healing journey.

The power of intention can serve as a powerful guiding force toward true healing and happiness. Intentionality is not just a floating thought; it is a deliberate and mindful choice to direct our energy and focus toward the values, aspirations, and experiences that align with our authentic selves.

Intention setting can be an invitation to cultivate a conscious and purposeful approach to each day, recognizing that our thoughts and actions shape the reality we experience.

I would like to invite you explore your intention for your healing journey. It might give you invaluable insights about yourself and your goals and values.

Here's how intention setting empowers us on our path to healing.

1. **Clarity and Focus**

   Intention setting allows us to sit a moment and clarify our goals. It gives us a possibility to focus our energy on what truly matters to us. In somatic therapy, setting clear intentions provides a roadmap for the healing journey, guiding individuals towards their desired outcomes.

2. **Alignment with Healing**

   By consciously setting intentions aligned with healing, individuals cultivate a sense of agency and empowerment over their healing process. Intention setting in somatic therapy enables individuals to establish a positive mindset and cultivate self-compassion, essential ingredients for healing.

3. **Mind-Body Connection**

   Intention setting can bridge the gap between our mind and body, fostering a deeper awareness of our physical and emotional experiences. In somatic therapy, setting intentions helps us connect with our bodily sensations, and helps to facilitate the release of stored trauma and promote overall wellbeing.

4. **Amplifying Resilience**

   Intention setting cultivates resilience. It can instill hope and optimism in us on our somatic therapy journey. Setting intentions to overcome challenges and embrace growth empowers us to navigate obstacles with courage and perseverance. (Yes, you are a superhero; you remember that, right?! Please keep it in mind, especially in tough moments.)

5. **Integration and Transformation**

   Intention setting serves as a catalyst for real integration and transformation in somatic therapy. By setting intentions aligned with personal growth and healing, we can pave the way for profound shifts in our inner landscape, leading to lasting change and real, authentic fulfillment.

In conclusion, intention setting is a powerful tool in the somatic therapy healing journey, empowering us to cultivate clarity, alignment, and resilience as we navigate our path to healing and beautiful transformation of our lives. By harnessing the power of intention, we can embark on a journey of self-discovery, growth, and holistic wellbeing.

What Actually Is Intention? Intention can be many things. It can be:

- An outcome you want
- Asking for insights or healing in certain areas of your life
- Hoping to see or develop some characteristics in yourself
- An experience in the session you wish to have

What an intention should not be:

- A requirement or demand
- An expectation

Once you set your intention, lovingly let go of it. This is the part where you set your trust in the experience. You have done your part and raked up for your end of the garden, so to speak.

Now, it's time to—gently—let go, trust the experience, and open yourself to what will arise.

WHAT DO INTENTIONS DO?

There are a number of uses that intentions have before, during, and after your healing journey.

THEY GUIDE AND HELP YOU TO "SHOW UP"

Setting an intention is the first step in really "showing up" for your healing process.

Intention informs your subconscious.

Through your intention, you can further assist this process by telling your body and mind, and especially your inner healing intelligence, what you think is most important to focus on right now.

Always remember your inner healing intelligence.

THEY GROUND AND RECENTER YOU

If at any point throughout your healing journey you feel challenged, unsure, or otherwise resistant to the content or nature of your experience, coming back to your intention can help to ground and recenter you on your journey.

It can help you make sense of the content of the experience in the moment, and it gives you an anchor, a point of rootedness to return to should you ever feel the need.

Cracking the code of our emotional, spiritual, and physical NOW is like having a treasure map to a better tomorrow. It's the launchpad for positive vibes, growth, and all-around awesomeness. Think of it as tuning into your internal GPS—understanding where you're at to chart the course for where you want to be.

So, ditch the autopilot, tap into your inner compass, and set sail for a brighter, better horizon.

Here we go.

WHAT IS YOUR GOAL/INTENTION WITH YOUR SOMATIC THERAPY JOURNEY?

Please sit with the intention for a moment. Something in the idea of somatic therapy invited you in, and when you reach out to that, it might give you valuable insights to explore your motivation and intention.

You can, if you like, take a moment to reflect these questions. Consider journaling, too.

What was it that drew you towards this book?

What can you make of the information you gave yourself in the previous question? Any surprises?

And some more: What can you make of the information you gave yourself in the previous page? Any surprises?

CHAPTER 1
INTRODUCTION TO SOMATIC THERAPY

"Traumatic events are almost impossible to put into words."
–Dr. Bessel van der Kolk

I remember him very clearly. He had mid-brown hair, friendly eyes, and he wasn't one of those people wanting to make noise about himself. On the contrary. There was something very earthly about him. That's the only word I feel describes him.

I had attended this seminar shortly after we had lost our child, and it was painful to be around people. I felt like I had to wear a happy mask. I don't even know why I felt that way. I guess because I thought that was expected. He used to be a high-end mathematician, working in various projects in the university world. Today he was walking in front of our university class, and saying, "I used to treat my body as just a carrying case for my brain, before I realized how beautiful all of it is connected."

It really hit me. I don't know how anyone could have said it more powerfully, and I realized my approach had pretty much been the same. Except my connection to my body had mainly been being worried if I had gained weight. (I would have hoped the world would have changed since then, but no, our young girls and ladies seem to have pretty much the same worries, if not even more intensive with the social media pressures and pleasing not only the people in the "real world," but also The Mightly Algorithm.)

That former mathematician and current life student changed my view for life.

Firstly, I started to pay attention that I actually had a body carrying my cortex.

Secondly, I started to note how I felt in various situations, and how I felt it in my body.

This was a totally new approach, and I can tell you, it took some getting used to.

I became a passionate searcher. I studied psychology even deeper. I read about different therapy modalities, mind-body connections through different lenses, breathing, yoga, meditation, trauma, trauma healing, trauma healing through different mind-body modalities, talking therapies, family dynamics, childhood trauma—basically everything I could find.

And—can you see the pattern?

I learned all I could, in my head.

Yes, I still was just in my head!

Just to show you how easy it is, to stay there:

One person who took me out of there, was my therapist. She was annoyingly calm, always, and she asked all the questions I didn't want anyone to ask.

She used to ask, for example, this: "Where do you feel it in your body?"

How should I know!

I learned a lot, and still I am on my journey. This lovely little hike called life is about learning, and healing, but mainly about finding the freedom and joy, don't you think?

When I began my studies in psychology, the common view was the brain was pretty much set after a certain age. (Yes, this was too long ago, in the early 90s, if you wonder.)

That sometimes lead even to a pretty hopeless world view: if you screwed up, you pretty much were doomed.

Now, thank goodness, the neuroscience understands, and all the research points to the direction neuroplasticity. That is the beautiful capacity to change our brain (and our mind, health, perception, beliefs, fears… to heal) no matter what age.

So, now, if you look at healing, you can also see it like this: even the (neuro)science supports your healing, my dear.

THE NEUROSCIENCE OF (SOMATIC) HEALING

"The mind/body connection is like a telephone line—many telephone lines, in fact, teeming with information. Small things like drinking an orange juice with pulp or eating an apple is being received like a telephone call to your genes. Every thought, everything you eat, every single little thing can tweak your genes' activity towards healing."

—Deepak Chopra

Our brain is an amazing organ. It just doesn't stop surprising me. The ability that our brain has to rewire and re-organize itself is simply amazing.
If you are anything like me, you ask: Where is the science in this? That's a good question and deserves an answer.

Research shows our brain can rewire itself, forming new neural pathways and connections, which is crucial for recovery from trauma. This can be done with the help of many modalities, also with somatic therapy.

Understanding neuroplasticity can help us understand the beautiful principles of healing and recovery from trauma-related conditions and guide us to… a better life, don't you think?

So, with somatic techniques, we can help rewire our neural pathways, also the ones associated with trauma. In the process, we can develop healthy and new responses to our emotional challenges and stressors, with a beautiful collaboration with our brain (and body).

Somatic therapy leverages neuroplasticity to facilitate healing from trauma by engaging our body's innate ability to adapt and change. Techniques such as mindfulness, breathwork, and body-centered exercises promote neuroplasticity by stimulating our brain's capacity for change and growth. By focusing on bodily sensations and experiences, somatic therapy encourages our brain to rewire maladaptive patterns associated with trauma, which can lead to our symptoms reducing and resilience increasing.

Doesn't this give a hopeful approach to healing?

As a counselor, I can also assure you, it happens. I have seen it happen to so many beautiful people in my therapy room. It can happen to you too.

Healing is possible, my dear, also from the neuroscience point of view. The science supports your healing.

SOMATIC THERAPY AT ITS VERY SIMPLEST

To put somatic therapy in its simplest form, we can view it like this:

Stage 1: We do the work.

Stage 2: We heal.

To put the goal the simplest: We move towards healthy wholeness. And then we repeat.

And everybody lived happily ever after. (Ish.)

So simple and neat, right?

THE ORIGINS OF SOMATIC THERAPY

"No matter where we are, the shadow that trots behind us is definitely four-footed."

—Clarissa Pinkaola Estes, Ph.D. From *Women Who Run With The Wolves*

Somatic therapy has its roots in various historical and theoretical frameworks that emphasize the connection between the body and the mind. Here is a brief overview:

1. **Wilhelm Reich and Body Armoring**

   Somatic therapy finds its beginnings in the work of Wilhelm Reich, a psychoanalyst who introduced the concept of "body armoring." Reich theorized that emotional experiences are stored in the body as muscular tension, leading to psychological and physical distress.

2. **Alexander Lowen and Bioenergetics**

   Building upon Reich's ideas, Alexander Lowen developed bioenergetics in the 1950s. Bioenergetics focuses on releasing physical tensions and emotional blockages through body-oriented techniques like breathing exercises, movement, and expressive therapies.

3. **Peter A. Levine and Somatic Experiencing**

In the late 20th century, Peter A. Levine developed somatic experiencing (SE) after observing how animals naturally recover from traumatic experiences. SE aims to heal trauma by addressing the body's physiological responses and restoring the nervous system's natural regulation. Levine wrote a gorgeous book, *Waking The Tiger*, which I'd recommend warmly as a read.

4. **Integration into Modern Psychotherapy**

Over time, somatic therapy has been integrated into various therapeutic modalities, such as somatic experiencing therapy, sensorimotor psychotherapy, and others. These approaches combine elements of neuroscience, psychology, and body-centered practices to address trauma, stress, and emotional wellbeing.

Somatic therapy's origins reflect a deep understanding of the interplay between our bodily sensations, emotions, and psychological wellbeing, opening the way for innovative approaches to healing and personal growth.

There is plenty of scientific research supporting the benefits of somatic therapy. For instance, studies suggest that somatic therapy may effectively reduce symptoms of post-traumatic stress disorder (PTSD), depression, and anxiety.

Research also indicates the effectiveness of somatic experiencing, a body-based trauma therapy, in addressing the physical symptoms of trauma.

Several studies demonstrate the positive effects, for example, of Eye Movement Desensitization and Reprocessing (EMDR), a type of somatic therapy, in treating psychological trauma. (This I would advise no one doing on their own, so my dear, please consider EMDR always only with a professional therapist.)

While I must say, somatic therapy shows promise, it's also good to be aware that more studies are needed to gain a deeper understanding of somatic therapy's potential advantages.

Overall, somatic therapy's effectiveness in treating various mental health conditions underscores its importance in holistic approaches to our psychological (and even holistic) wellbeing. Further research can provide deeper insights into its mechanisms and efficacy.

HOW SOMATIC THERAPY DIFFERS FROM TALK THERAPY

Sometimes talking (therapy) just isn't enough. I know this from my personal experience. I went to psychotherapy twice a week for four years, and still I felt something was missing.

Then I read Levine's book *Waking The Tiger* and realized that was the part I needed.

The beauty about somatic therapy is you don't necessarily have to revisit the trauma in any way, it just helps to release the marks of the trauma that has been stored in your body. I love Levine's work. I am so happy I found his book, and I recommend it to you too if you want to learn more about how trauma and the body are connected.

Levine's book opened so much to me. I went to all kinds of courses. I went to yoga, yoga guidance, TRE where I literally was shaking my a*s off (and released so much tension, stress, and trauma), I went running, and I went walking.

I want to add also: I don't want to say talk therapies do not work. On the contrary, there is plenty of scientific proof it does work, but sometimes we need more than that, something different.

We are all different and need different things. We might even need different things in different phases in our lives. I would like to give you a brief overview of how the traditional "top-down" talk therapy approach differs from the "bottom-up" somatic modalities.

1. **Focus**

   - **Talk Therapy (also known as "Top-Down Therapy")**

     Talk therapy, as we might guess, primarily focuses on verbal communication and cognitive exploration to understand emotions and behaviors. This can also be very effective when done right.

   - **Somatic Therapy (also known as "Bottom-Up Therapy")**

     Emphasizes the body's sensations, movements, and experiences to address psychological issues, trauma, and stress. Somatic therapy aims to connect the body and mind and provide holistic wellbeing.

2. **Techniques**

   - **Talk Therapy**

     Uses conversation, reflection, and analysis to explore thoughts, feelings, and behaviors.

   - **Somatic Therapy**

     Incorporates body-centered techniques such as breathwork, movement, touch, and mindfulness to ease and release tension, trauma, and stress stored in the body.

3. **Goals**

   - **Talk Therapy**

Aims to gain insight, develop coping strategies, and promote psychological wellbeing through conscious awareness.

- **Somatic Therapy**

  Seeks to regulate the nervous system and release physical tension, process trauma, and integrate the mind-body connection for a holistic healing experience.

Somatic therapy and talk therapy offer distinct approaches to mental health treatment, with somatic therapy uniquely focusing on the body's role in emotional processing and healing.

FORMS OF SOMATIC THERAPY

Somatic therapy comes in many forms, which the easiest forms can be, in my opinion, practiced with a guided workbook like this. However, there are some forms which I wouldn't advise you to try at home.

Some Somatic Therapy Techniques

- Breathing exercises
- Grounding
- Mindfulness
- Movement therapies
- Touch and bodywork
- Dancing
- Resourcing

TRE® (TENSION AND TRAUMA RELEASING EXERCISES)

I love TRE®. I have found deep healing through it personally, and I have been fortunate to see many of my clients transform beautifully practicing TRE® has helped their nervous systems and bodies to return to a calm, healthy baseline.

(*Homeostasis,* again, a word crafted from ancient Greek, which is the beautiful state of balance.)

TRE® was developed by David Berceli, Ph.D., who is an international expert in the areas of conflict resolution and trauma intervention. TRE® safely activates a natural reflex mechanism of shaking or vibrating that releases muscular tension, calming down the nervous system.

TRE®—OR JUST SIMPLY SHAKING—IN SOMATIC THERAPY

1. **Overview**

   TRE®, or Tension & Trauma Releasing Exercises, is a technique within somatic therapy that focuses on releasing deep muscular patterns of stress, tension, and trauma.

2. **Polyvagal Theory**

   TRE® is informed by the polyvagal theory, which explains how the autonomic nervous system responds to stress and trauma. When we activate the body's natural tremor mechanism, TRE aims to regulate the nervous system and promote relaxation.

3. **Body-Centered Approach**

   TRE® recognizes the interconnection between our body and emotions. It underlines that the body holds emotional experiences, and when we release physical tension, our emotional healing can occur.

4. **Trauma Healing**

   TRE® can be particularly effective in trauma recovery. It can offer a gentle and non-invasive way to address traumatic experiences. Yes, through the release of physical tension, our trauma symptoms may reduce, and resilience may increase.

5. **Stress Reduction**

Beyond trauma, TRE® can also be beneficial for stress reduction and overall wellbeing. Through TRE® exercises, we can find relaxation, improve sleep quality, and enhance our ability to cope with daily stressors.

6. **Differences from Somatic Experiencing**

While both TRE® and Somatic Experiencing aim to address trauma and stress-related issues, they are based on slightly different techniques and approaches. TRE® primarily focuses on activating the body's natural tremor response, while somatic experiencing emphasizes tracking bodily sensations and titrating traumatic experiences.

Overall, TRE® can be a practical and accessible method for releasing stress and trauma from the body.

There are also other deep methods, which I do not recommend doing at home, like EMDR therapy (Eye Movement Desensitization and Reprocessing), which can be a very effective therapeutic tool, but from my perspective, it should always only be done with a skilled and professional therapist. EMDR therapy is *a treatment for conditions involving traumatic memories, and precisely because of involving the traumatic memories, please only do it with a professional who you trust. Promise me?*

EMDR done professionally has shown indications to be very effective, and it can reshape the past events and give a lot of emotional space. EMDR can help build connections between the physical body and the psychological mind, and reduce stress response.

But again, my dear, please seek professional support, if you are interested in exploring EMDR therapy.

SOME KEY TERMS

First, before we dive in, it is beneficial to go through a few key terms that we are going to be using quite a lot in this book, and you will benefit knowing what we mean by them in these pages.

MIND-BODY CONNECTION

We usually are more than our outer layer of our brain which we often would love to be. We also are more than this leather bag we live in. Our culture may push us in the other direction, and we might lose the connection between those two when we try so hard to concentrate on one or the other. Many of us have personal experience of that.

The body-mind connection usually refers to the intricate relationship between our physical health and our mental and emotional states. It acknowledges that our thoughts, emotions, and beliefs can influence our biological functioning, and conversely, physical health can impact mental and emotional wellbeing and vice versa. This interconnectedness suggests that what happens in the mind can affect the body—and the other way around. Understanding and nurturing this connection can lead to holistic approaches to health and wellness, emphasizing the importance of addressing both mental and physical aspects of our wellbeing.

So, when we find the harmonious connection between the two, our wellbeing usually improves.

SOMATIC EXPERIENCING THERAPY

Somatic experiencing therapy, also known as somatic therapy, focuses on treating mental and emotional health issues by addressing bodily sensations and experiences. It recognizes the interconnection between the mind and body and aims to release tension and trauma stored in the body to promote healing.

SOMATIC AWARENESS

As you may guess, this term refers to the ability to notice and understand bodily sensations, feelings, and movements. Developing somatic awareness is a fundamental aspect of somatic therapy, as it allows individuals to recognize and process emotional and physical experiences stored in the body.

PENT-UP EMOTIONS

Pent-up emotions are feelings that have been suppressed or stored in the body without being fully expressed or processed. Somatic therapy can help us release these emotions by accessing and addressing them through bodily sensations and movements. This can be stress management, movement techniques, emotional release, and other methods, like we will guide you through later in this book.

CHAPTER 2
UNDERSTANDING TRAUMA

"Your trauma is not your fault, but healing is your ~~responsibility~~ **right.***"*

—Unknown

You might have seen this beautiful quote before, emphasizing your responsibility in trauma healing. But I would change the word "responsibility" to the word "right."

You have the **right** to heal.

You have the **right** to be happy and enjoy life.

Remember, you are not alone. We all struggle—every single one of us have trauma, in different degrees. You are *allowed* to struggle; not everything has to be neat and perfect!

Your inner wisdom guided you to somatic therapy, and you were brave enough to listen to it. I think you should, once again, praise yourself for that.

Now we will take a closer look at trauma and trauma healing, so you can form an understanding about your life and trauma, and especially healing with somatic therapy.

UNDERSTANDING TRAUMA AND TRAUMA HEALING IN SOMATIC THERAPY

What Is Trauma?

One word that we have been seeing and hearing about a LOT on the internet is trauma. Everyone talks about it, and it can have different connotations in different situations and even different people.

Many associate the word "trauma" to extreme conditions, like wars, and while they usually are very traumatizing, trauma can be so many things. It usually refers to the emotional, psychological, and physical responses to an extremely distressing or disturbing event(s) that overwhelm our ability to cope. It can result from various experiences, including but not limited to accidents, abuse, violence, natural disasters, or sudden loss. Trauma often leads to feelings of intense fear, helplessness, and horror. It can have lasting effects on our mental, emotional, and physical wellbeing. These effects may include symptoms such as intrusive memories, flashbacks, nightmares, anxiety, depression, and difficulty regulating emotions.

We *all* have trauma in some degree, in my opinion. It's kind of part of the deal on our hike on this planet called life, inside our funny little leather bags.

The other, totally different, question is, do we have to *suffer* from our traumas, and if so, *how much*?

I'm guessing those are questions you have asked, too, since you are here with us. (We love that you are here with us!)

The short answer is: no, we absolutely do *not* have to suffer from our traumas.
The long answer is a bit more complicated, since it involves the different types of traumas, and the depths and complexities of them, the unconscious parts of them, and so forth.

So I like the short answer better, and even though we can't totally ignore the long answer, we can still focus on the healing.

Why?

Because life is so much more fulfilling and fun on the other side of trauma. It's light, and it has light, and it's… beautiful.

WHAT TRAUMA IS AND WHAT IT IS NOT

Sometimes it´s hard to separate which is normal wear and tear, and which is trauma. I would say, like I wrote earlier, trauma is an overwhelming experience that we can not cope with.

One thing important to know, is that trauma is not a disease. Trauma expert, Levine, defines it as *dis-ease*.

Also, trauma is not a psychical disorder, neither a physiological one. Trauma symptoms are a perfectly natural reaction to a distressing event where we may have felt overwhelmed, afraid, or helpless. It's a natural response, my dear.

Common trauma symptoms might be some of these:

- Flashbacks: vivid and distressing recollections of the traumatic event.
- Nightmares and difficulty sleeping: disturbing dreams related to the traumatic experience.
- Anxiety: Persistent feelings of apprehension, nervousness, or fear. Feeling on edge, jumpiness or startling easily.
- Avoidance: efforts to avoid reminders of the traumatic event.
- Helplessness.
- Dissociation, emotional numbness, social withdrawal, loss of interest in activities.
- Changes in attention, concentration, and memory retrieval.

- Changes in behavior, attitude, worldview.
- Difficulty functioning.
- Denial, or refusing to believe that the trauma occurred.
- Anger.
- Hypervigilance: heightened state of alertness, always scanning for danger.
- Emotional numbness: feeling detached or disconnected from others.
- Irritability: increased irritability, anger, or outbursts.
- Sexual dysfunction, difficulty becoming aroused, or difficulty reaching orgasm.
- Intrusive thoughts: unwanted and distressing thoughts or memories about the trauma.
- Guilt or shame: feelings of responsibility or self-blame for the traumatic event.
- Social withdrawal: avoidance of social activities or isolation from others.
- Sleep disturbances: difficulty falling asleep or staying asleep, nightmares.
- Physical symptoms: Headaches, stomachaches, or other physical discomfort related to stress. Increased heart rate, body aches or pains, tense muscles, fatigue.
- Difficulty concentrating: inability to focus or concentrate on tasks.
- Startle response: easily startled or frightened by sudden noises or movements.
- Changes in appetite: eating too much or too little as a coping mechanism.
- Substance abuse: increased use of alcohol or drugs to cope with emotions.
- Depression: persistent feelings of sadness, hopelessness, or despair.
- Relationship problems: strained relationships with family, friends, or colleagues.

- Loss of interest: lack of interest in activities once enjoyed.
- Suicidal thoughts: thoughts of death or suicide as a way to escape the pain.

DIFFERENT TYPES OF TRAUMAS

We are all on this same hike called life, and it's important to understand that trauma can have an impact on people of any age, be it a child or an adult. We also may experience situations and traumas differently. Even the same events may affect us differently.

Let's also define trauma as shortly as we can: trauma is an emotional response triggered by a distressing event or series of events.

It's also beneficial to understand there are different types of most common traumas.

1. **Acute Trauma** usually results from a single stressful event, like accidents or natural disasters.

2. **Chronic Trauma** is more persistent exposure to stressful situations over time, such as ongoing abuse or living in a war zone.

3. **Complex Trauma** arises from prolonged exposure to multiple traumatic events, often during childhood, and may lead to complex post-traumatic stress disorder (CPTSD).

4. **Secondary Trauma** may occur when experiencing indirectly by witnessing or hearing about traumatic events happening to others, affecting healthcare workers, first responders, or family members of trauma survivors.

5. **Vicarious Trauma** is similar to secondary trauma, and it can occur when individuals absorb the traumatic experiences of others they care for, such as therapists or caregivers.

6. **Developmental Trauma** is experienced during critical developmental stages, impacting psychological and emotional development, and often may lead to long-term effects on behavior and mental health.

7. **Cumulative Trauma** can result from the accumulation of various stressful events or adverse experiences over time, significantly affecting an individual's wellbeing and functioning.

Post-traumatic stress disorder (PTSD) and complex PTSD (CPTSD) are specific types of trauma-related disorders, characterized by intense stress reactions following exposure to traumatic events.

HOW TRAUMA AFFECTS THE BODY

I will tell you this. Our body is not just the passive storage space for trauma—our trauma actually *affects our body constantly*.

So, it's not just in our heads. Trauma *does* affect the body. There are so many studies done, we can say it with total confidence.

(The beauty is, we can also *reduce* the affects *through the body*, for example somatic therapy!)

You might be familiar with these common symptoms, how trauma (and stress) affects the body.

HOW DO WE KNOW IF WE HAVE TRAUMA?

Well, for example these symptoms might indicate we may be suffering from trauma:

1. **Physical Symptoms**

   Trauma can lead to physical ailments such as headaches, body aches, and fatigue. There can be stomach issues, sleeping problems, muscle tension and pain, increased heart rate and blood pressure, hormone imbalances, skin conditions, compromised reproductive health, and so many others.

2. Somatic Responses

Somatic responses to trauma include shaking, sweating, and changes in appetite.

3. Arousal Dysregulation

Traumatized individuals may experience hyperarousal (e.g., heightened senses, hypervigilance) or hypoarousal (e.g., numbness, dissociation) and even hypervigilance. Hypervigilance means you will feel you're on high alert and on a constant lookout for any threats. (Was that a tiger in the bush?!) It is an exhausting state mentally and physically. Trust me, I used to be that. (And I am not so much anymore, so my dear, there is hope. There always is hope!)

4. Immobilization Defenses

Some may exhibit immobilizing defenses like freezing, characterized by a sense of paralysis and hyperalert senses.

5. Memory and Cognitive Issues

Trauma can impair memory, concentration, and cognitive functioning. Emotional dysregulation like anger, mood swings, and irritability.

6. Chronic Health Conditions

Prolonged trauma (and stress) exposure may increase the risk of weakened immune system function and chronic health conditions, such as cardiovascular diseases and autoimmune disorders.

TRAUMA RELEASE

Somatic therapy aims to facilitate the release of trauma stored in the body's tissues and nervous system. Through various techniques, such as breathing exercises, movement, and touch, individuals can discharge stored traumatic energy and restore a sense of safety and equilibrium.

THE WINDOW OF TOLERANCE

We all have our window of tolerance, whether we are aware of it or not. It refers to the range of emotional and physiological states in which we feel comfortable and can function effectively.

1. **Hyperarousal and Hypoarousal**: When we are within our window of tolerance, we can navigate life's challenges without becoming overwhelmed or dissociated. Hyperarousal occurs when stress levels are too high, leading to anxiety or panic, while hypoarousal involves feeling emotionally numb or shut down.

2. **Importance in Somatic Therapy**

   Somatic exercises can help us identify our window of tolerance and develop skills to expand it. Techniques such as mindfulness, breathwork, and body awareness exercises aim to regulate arousal levels and promote resilience for us to find life more... well, not only tolerable, but joyful and fulfilling.

3. **Trauma and the Window of Tolerance**

   Individuals with a history of trauma often have a narrower window of tolerance, making them more susceptible to dysregulation. But read this: somatic therapy aims to offer tools to gently expand this window, allowing for increased capacity to tolerate distress.

Understanding and working within the window of tolerance is very important in somatic therapy, strengthening our ability to regulate emotions, manage stress, and grow our resilience.

That's why I have designed this program for you to have alternatives each day to choose the option so you can stay in your own window of tolerance.

ARE WE ENTITLED TO HAVE TRAUMA?

Then there comes the big question regarding whether we are entitled to have traumatic experiences. Does someone have it even worse?

I have seen people survive in absolutely terrible situations, barely making it alive, and thinking some people have it even worse. They feel they are not entitled to have a trauma because someone might be in war or in the middle of a natural disaster or massacre.

Like Susan, who came to me. She had been visiting me twice a week for some time. She was in her fifties, working as a director in an advertising agency. She paid a lot of attention to her wellbeing and studied a lot about it. She told me she had found her childhood love again, horses, and she'd started horseback riding again. In one lesson she'd done showjumping, and her horse had tripped in the jump, and in a split second, Susan had fallen with the horse from a gallop, face first. Susan got up (she was able to get up) and checked the horse was ok. She didn't really understand what had happened. Everything around her felt like it happened far away, like she was in some kind of bubble where all the sounds and visuals were funny. (She was in shock.) She spit something from her mouth; it appeared to be a piece of a tooth. Also, she got blood on her hand when she touched her face.

"But this was just a riding accident. Some people have it so much worse," she said to me when I asked how she felt about the accident now.
(What happened after the fall, I will tell you later.)

This is absolutely *human*.

But my dear, trauma is a trauma. It is something that has happened to us (or even near us) *that has been overwhelming to us.* Trauma doesn't ask if someone has it worse; trauma is a response that we have instinctively, without a choice.

So please, if you have these feelings, try to put them aside. **Try to see yourself worthy to receive the guidance and exercises in this book.** This book has been written especially for you.

THE BEAUTIFUL BENEFITS OF DEALING WITH OUR TRAUMA

Many of us, quite rightly, feel a little intimidated with the idea of heading on the path of facing our traumas.

If we are brave enough to step on the path of dealing with our traumas—you clearly are—it can lead to so many gorgeous benefits. Most of the time, it's a journey that teaches so much about ourselves, our strengths, and wisdom. Often, it helps develop deeper and healthier relationships and healthier boundaries.

Even with a risk of going a little outside of our somatic therapy concept, I want to share this spiritual thought with you. *Author, researcher, and lecturer Dr.* Joe Dispenza words it beautifully in Jay Shetty's podcast. Dispenza talks about people who have meditated in his workshops and have achieved a very deep altered state where they "connect" with their higher power, they look back on their lives and would not change a single thing, because they know *all the difficulties brought them to this moment.*

In my opinion, we'd be so much better off if we were able not to judge our traumas, our lives, and our reactions. I hope Dispenza's observation can also give comfort to you. (It certainly has brought comfort for me, both as a professional but also as a fellow traveler.)

SOME BENEFITS OF TRAUMA WORK:

1. **Increased Resilience**

Dealing with trauma can foster resilience, enabling us to bounce back from adversity with newfound strength.

2. **Personal Growth**

Through the process of healing, we often experience profound personal growth, gaining deeper insights into ourselves and our capabilities.

3. **Enhanced Empathy**

Having faced our own struggles, trauma survivors often develop a heightened sense of empathy and compassion towards others who are going through difficult times.

4. **Improved Relationships**

Addressing trauma can lead to healthier relationships as we learn to communicate effectively, set healthier boundaries, and cultivate intimacy.

5. **Positive Life Changes**

Many of us find that dealing with trauma prompts positive changes in our lives, such as pursuing new interests, reevaluating priorities, and fostering a greater sense of purpose.

UNDERSTANDING THE ROLE OF THE NERVOUS SYSTEM IN TRAUMA HEALING AND SOMATIC THERAPY

"The mind and body communicate constantly. What you think, feel, and believe affects your body, and how your body feels affects your mind."
— Unknown

First, we will dive into the basics to help you understand the world of somatic therapy we are about to step in.

The word "somatic" originates from Ancient Greek—of course, like every civilized word does!—and to be more exact, from the word "sōmatikós," which means "bodily" or "of the body." The term "somatic" has been used historically to refer to the material body, distinct from other important concepts such as the soul, spirit, or mind.

Our body and mind are in constant communication. If you want proof of that, I'll demonstrate it to you. It will only take a moment.

All you really need to do is to close your eyes, and think about a lemon. Think about the color, how it feels in your hand, and how it tastes. Then open your eyes.

Did you taste the lemon? Was your mouth watering? Did you smell the lemon?

Or did you feel the weight of the lemon in your hand?

Your mind has incredible power, and it does communicate with your body all the time, whether you are aware of it or not.

Trauma affects our nervous system, sometimes very deep, influencing how we perceive and respond to the world around us. Somatic therapy aims to recognize the intricate connection between trauma and the nervous system, offering a beautiful, holistic approach to healing. Here's how the nervous system affects trauma recovery in somatic therapy:

1. **Fight, Flight, Freeze Response**

   When faced with trauma, the autonomic nervous system triggers the instinctual fight, flight, or freeze response. Somatic therapy can help us regulate these responses, promoting a sense of safety and security. Doesn't it sound wonderful? I, personally, have found this the most comforting and healing part of somatic therapy.

2. **Hyperarousal and Hypoarousal**

Trauma can lead to states of hyperarousal (excessive vigilance) or hypoarousal (numbing and disconnection). Somatic interventions aim to balance these states, restoring equilibrium to the nervous system. The balance, my dear!

3. **Interoception and Emotional Regulation**

Interoception, the ability to sense internal bodily states, is often impaired in trauma survivors. Somatic therapy fosters interoceptive awareness, facilitating emotional regulation and the processing of traumatic experiences.

4. **The Polyvagal Theory**

Somatic therapy draws on the principles of the polyvagal theory, which aims to explain the role of the vagus nerve in regulating social engagement, stress responses, and relaxation. By engaging the vagus nerve through somatic techniques, we may access states of safety and connection.

5. **Embodied Healing**

Somatic therapy emphasizes holistic embodied healing, recognizing that trauma is stored not only in the mind but also in the body. Through mindful awareness of bodily sensations and movement practices, we can release that stored trauma and restore our vitality, joy, and mind-body-connection.

By addressing the nervous system's intricate responses to trauma, somatic therapy aims to offer a beautiful path toward profound healing, resilience, joy, and happiness.

UNDERSTANDING THE POLYVAGAL THEORY DEEPER

Polyvagal theory gives us tools to understand how our nervous system works.

Just under the surface of our conscious awareness, we have a powerful machine working constantly to keep us safe and alive. To keep us in balance, *homeostasis* (again, another word from ancient Greek!). This machine works without our input, autonomically.

Yes, this is called our autonomic nervous system, which is formed from sympathetic and parasympathetic states.

To understand this, we need to take a look at polyvagal theory, which was coined by Stephen Porges, as well the term *neuroception*, which we all (mammals) have kind of as a built-in special equipment. For a short definition of neuroception: it means we all have a lovely built-in scanner inside us, constantly keeping an eye on our surroundings to gather information and evaluate if we are safe or in danger.

Our nervous systems have three very different states, depending how we perceive the surroundings. (Note: I literally mean *how we perceive the surroundings*, not how the surroundings *actually are*.)

Let's take a look at Amy. She is on a peaceful walk in the park she knows very well. She absolutely loves morning walks, and on top of all that: it's spring. If we take a look at her physics, her heart rate is regulated, she feels safe and happy, active and engaged. Her nervous system is in a parasympathetic state: her neuroception is in a ventral vagal state, meaning safe and social.

When we are in a ventral vagal, parasympathetic state, we are grounded, joyful, mindful, curious, compassionate, and empathetic.

Suddenly, Amy hears a siren. She sees a police car. She immediately becomes alert. Her *sympathetic nervous system* activates, her heart starts racing, her breath becomes shallow, she gets anxious, and she has a surge of adrenaline. She is in a state of fight-or-flight. The world for Amy now feels like a dangerous place.

The police car drives away, and eventually Amy is able to calm down back to the safe feeling, ventral vagal state. (It's also viewed as rest and digest, or *homeostasis,* meaning balanced state.)

On the way home Amy sees her ex who has had a lot of emotional regulation issues and occasionally been abusive. Amy's breath gets shallow again, and her energy gets very low. She feels disconnected and even numb, hopeless, alone, and foggy. This is yet another neuroception named dorsal vagal state, where Amy has shut down and dissociated as a survival mechanism.

The polyvagal theory offers us a neurophysiological framework to help to understand our actions are *automatic.* Amy absolutely did not make a conscious decision to make her heart rate go up (or down), she didn't consciously alter her breathing—it all came as an automatic response.

(In fact, we wouldn't even have time to regulate our responses, even if we wanted to, since our nervous system is reacting instinctively, even before we consciously think about our reactions.)

The polyvagal theory **suggests that the evolution of the mammalian autonomic nervous system provides the neuro-physiological substrates for adaptive behavioral strategies**. This comes from our early reptile brain, the very core of our nervous system.

This all comes from the early dawn of mammalian design. You can imagine, as Levine describes in his book *Waking The Tiger*, an impala on a savanna, attacked by a cheetah. As soon as, or even a split second before, the teeth and claws touch, the impala seems to drop dead. This is an example of an extreme, instinctive behavior protecting us in life-threatening circumstances.

(It might be nicer to be eaten by a cheetah or a tiger being totally numb, don't you think?)

Our neuroception is constantly scanning our surroundings. Even when we meet someone new, we unconsciously scan for clues as to whether we are safe or in danger with that person nearby.

The nerve connecting our body's reaction with our scans is the vagus nerve, which literally means "wondering." Let's get to know this superhero nerve a little better.

SO, WHAT IS THE FAMOUS VAGUS NERVE?

In Latin the term "vagus" means wondering, which gives a good picture of what it (quite literally!) is.

The vagus nerve, also known as the **tenth cranial nerve, cranial nerve X**, or simply **CN X,** is the longest cranial nerve in our body and it literally "wanders" from the brain to the body and back. It extends from the brainstem down into the abdomen. It is formed by a complex network of fibers originating from the medulla oblongata in the brainstem.

Simpler, please?

Ok. The vagus nerve quite literally connects brain stems through our heart, lungs, digestive system, liver, gallbladder, spleen, pancreas and kidneys.

The vagus nerve literally is the rock star, the key player, when we aim to heal from our trauma. We need to retrain our vagus nerve, literally reset our nervous system. In somatic therapy we have tools to help build *vagal tone*, strengthening our capacity to switch from fight-or-flight (or freeze) into rest-and-digest.

When we activate the vagus nerve, we stimulate the parasympathetic nervous system and we can rewire our neural pathways towards… are you ready… calm, relaxed, compassionate, and creative states. In rest-and-digest we are able to feel safe, relax, learn, *connect*, digest our food, *love*. We are able to shift our attention from outer constant threats to… healing.

(By the way. Take a look at television news, or even better, social media platforms. Which nervous system state do you think they are built on?)

FUNCTIONS OF THE VAGUS NERVE:

1. **Autonomic Functions**

   Regulates various autonomic functions, such as heart rate, digestion, respiratory rate, and blood pressure.

2. **Parasympathetic Nervous System**

   Controls the parasympathetic nervous system, which is responsible for the body's rest-and-digest response.

3. **Sensory Functions**

   Provides sensory information from the organs of the chest and abdomen to the brain, including taste sensation from the back of the tongue.

4. **Motor Functions**

   Supplies motor fibers to muscles of the pharynx, larynx, and soft palate, influencing speech and swallowing.

POLYVAGAL THEORY, VAGUS NERVE, AND TRAUMA

Here is another very important thing to understand about our nervous system states.

A normal person is pretty freely able to switch from a parasympathetic to sympathetic and back.

We, who have experienced trauma, have a higher risk to get stuck on the constant sympathetic or dorsal vagal state.

(I know this. I have been on a sympathetic state since… well, probably from the womb. I have literally had to learn to teach my body I am safe when I am safe, and it's been a learning process.)

Karen was bullied in her work in her twenties. She was working while studying, and the culture at her workplace was very toxic. First, she tried to stand up for herself. That didn't work, and the bullying continued. Karen's fight-or-flight response didn't work, so her nervous system switched to dorsal vagal shutdown, which was her last option.

Now when we look at Karen's situation through the lens of polyvagal theory, we understand trauma impacted Karen's ability to regulate her nervous system. Her natural pattern of social connection has been switched to protection.

In short, Karen's nervous system is now wired for danger and threat, not safety and connection. She views the world through a dorsal vagal state; her ability to scan her surroundings has become disturbed. In other words, her neuroception is faulty leading her to overestimate danger and threat and miss the cues for safety and connection.

Trauma(s) has shaped Karen's nervous system. These wounds require healing, with a healing relationship, where Karen can learn to trust people.

As you can see, this is a paradox. Karen—as we all do—needs a connection to heal, but at the same time connection feels dangerous.

In these kinds of situations talk therapy can help to gain trust in other people by *co-regulating* by the therapist, giving safe clues, reassuring Karen the environment and the connection is safe. Often combined with somatic therapy the help may increase deeper healing.

Our society doesn't make it easy for us to stay in a parasympathetic, rest-and-digest state either. When our neuroception gets bombed with social media notifications, street ads, two-minute videos, tons of them, neon lights, motorways, time lapses, it often means we trying to survive in constant fight-or-flight.

Do you see the connection with stomach issues, and other chronic diseases?

By the way, our nervous system can *only be in one state at a time.*

When I realized this, I turned off all of my notifications, set a screen time limit for myself and disconnected from social media debates.

I can tell you; it has helped enormously.

HOW IS THE VAGUS NERVE RELATED TO OUR FOCUS, SOMATIC THERAPY?

Well, in many ways.

1. **Body-Mind Connection**

   Somatic therapy recognizes the bidirectional communication between the body and the mind. Our vagus nerve plays a key role in this two-way communication.

2. **Regulation of the Nervous System**

Somatic therapy techniques aim to regulate the nervous system, promoting relaxation and reducing stress. The vagus nerve is strongly involved in the body's stress response and relaxation processes.

3. **Emotional Processing**

Somatic therapy facilitates the releasing and processing of emotions stored in our body. By engaging the vagus nerve through somatic techniques, we can access and integrate emotional experiences more effectively.

The vagus nerve's role in regulating bodily functions and its connection to emotional processing make it an important aspect of somatic therapy, which focuses on healing trauma and promoting overall wellbeing through body-centered approaches.

Remember Susan, who fell with her horse? Susan was clearly affected by the riding accident, to the point that she felt a little ashamed to even talk about it. She felt there were so many people out there in desperate conditions, so, "Who am I to complain about my first world problems?" she said.

I felt it was not necessary for her to relive her accident in any way, and we started doing somatic experiencing exercises. Shaking exercises really seemed to help her. Every time I guided her—through certain exercises—to shake her body, she became so relaxed and so... *present* in her body. She was so *present* in the moment. I could see it in her, it was so beautiful. After 10 minutes of shaking, she became so relaxed, her breathing was calm, deep and... again, relaxed. She was attentive but so calm.

"I feel so... safe!" she said sounding a little surprised.

Then she remembered something. "OMG, this is what I did after the fall, too!" (She did not go to the doctor for a checkup, which I would have strongly advised her to do.)

She explained, she had taken her horse up and taken off the gear, then she had taken her horse back to the arena which was empty, and she had let her horse free.

"Then I went, for some reason, by the side of the arena and sat down." She then said she had started to shake uncontrollably, and she'd burst into tears. The horse came to stand beside her.

"There I sat on the sand of the arena, with the beautiful horse soul by my side, and I cried and cried. I couldn't stop it!"

She didn't remember how long she had been there with her horse. She thought it might have been an hour or even two.

"And after that I felt so much better. My horse stood by my side the whole time."

(A side note: This is why we also have animals working with therapists. Animals have unbelievably beautiful, infinite capacity to help us, on so many levels.)

"My horse had herself just experienced the same accident, and there she stood, right beside me, the whole time."

Somatic therapy often integrates polyvagal theory principles to help regulate the nervous system and promote safety. Somatic therapy may introduce exercises such as grounding techniques, breathwork, and gentle movements to nurture a sense of safety and connection, aligning with polyvagal theory's emphasis on social engagement and physiological regulation.

In summary, while polyvagal theory provides a neurobiological framework for understanding responses to stress and trauma, somatic therapy aims to apply this knowledge practically, using body-centered techniques to help us heal and regulate.

THE BEAUTIFUL BENEFITS OF SOMATIC THERAPY

If (somatic) therapy can be messy and hard, why do it?

—Because of the beautiful benefits, my dear.

Many times we think just brushing our problems under the carpet will help, and it might, for some time. But—unfortunately—only for some time. (Believe me, I used to be an expert in this field.)

After a while the past traumas will start popping on the surface, and they won't be pretty. That's why I so admire your courage to enter this healing path, even when it's not always easy.

Just to keep you motivated, I wanted to quickly list some of the benefits of somatic therapy.

The most beautiful benefit of somatic therapy, in my opinion and based on my experience, is that it can work gorgeously especially with trauma, in a way where we can free ourselves from stored tension in our bodies and wounds without having to necessarily revisit the painful event(s). Our body is so amazing it can release our pain without having to include the mind and the memories.

Personally, this is the main reason, after that speaker in that seminar helped me to understand I was more than just my brain and the brain-holding-carrier, I have since then used somatic methods to heal myself, and I can tell you, it works beautifully.

Of course, sometimes somatic therapy might help even more when combined with talk therapy. It's always a matter of the personal path that can provide the most support.

30 BENEFITS OF SOMATIC THERAPY

1. Can alleviate symptoms of PTSD

Somatic therapy can provide relief from PTSD symptoms by addressing underlying trauma and promoting healing. (We like that, don't we!)

2. Can reduce anxiety

Through somatic techniques, individuals can learn to calm their nervous system, reducing feelings of anxiety and promoting relaxation.

3. Can manage depression

Somatic therapy can offer tools to manage depression by integrating body awareness and emotional processing.

4. Can release pent-up emotions

By focusing on bodily sensations, somatic therapy can help individuals release stored emotions, leading to emotional relief.

5. Can restore the body's equilibrium

Somatic therapy is known to aid in restoring balance to the body's systems, promoting overall wellbeing and stability.

6. Can enhance emotional regulation

Through somatic practices, we can develop skills to regulate our emotions more effectively. (Very good skill to have, I might add.)

7. Can promote self-awareness

Somatic therapy can cultivate self-awareness by helping us connect with our bodily sensations and emotional experiences. (Again, we are mind-body creatures, not either/or.)

8. **Can improve body image**

By fostering acceptance and connection with the body, somatic therapy can improve body image and self-esteem.

9. **May increase relaxation**

Somatic techniques can induce relaxation responses in the body, promoting a sense of calm and tranquility. (This one I love!)

10. **Can support stress management skills**

Somatic therapy can also equip individuals with effective strategies to manage and cope with stressors in daily life.

11. **Can help cultivate mindfulness**

Through mindful awareness of bodily sensations, somatic therapy can cultivate present-moment awareness and mindfulness.

12. **May foster self-confidence**

Somatic therapy can empower us to trust our bodily experiences, leading to increased self-confidence.

13. **Can improve sleep quality**

By reducing physiological arousal and promoting relaxation, somatic therapy can improve sleep patterns and quality.

14. **May enhance interpersonal relationships**

Somatic therapy can foster deeper connections and communication skills, leading to more fulfilling relationships.

15. **May decrease chronic pain**

Somatic therapy can address the physical and emotional components of chronic pain, reducing its intensity and frequency.

16. May improve communication skills

By promoting body awareness and emotional expression, somatic therapy can enhance communication abilities.

17. Can strengthen resilience

Somatic therapy can build resilience by teaching us to adapt to stressors and challenges more effectively.

18. Can support addiction recovery

Somatic therapy can aid in addiction recovery by addressing underlying trauma and promoting holistic healing.

19. May enhance body awareness

Somatic therapy can increase body awareness, helping us firstly recognize and secondly respond to physical and emotional cues.

20. Can reduce muscle tension

Through relaxation techniques, somatic therapy can reduce muscle tension and promotes physical relaxation.

21. May improve digestion

Somatic therapy can positively impact digestion by reducing stress and promoting relaxation in the body. When we can switch from a fight-or-flight response to a relaxed state, our digestion is able to function how it's supposed to.

22. May boost immune function

By reducing stress levels and promoting overall wellbeing, somatic therapy can really support a healthy immune system.

23. Can increase energy levels

Somatic therapy can revitalize the body and mind, leading to increased energy levels and vitality.

24. Can promote overall wellbeing

Somatic therapy can enhance overall wellbeing by addressing the interconnectedness of the body and mind.

25. May enhance body-mind connection

Somatic therapy can strengthen the connection between the body and mind, promoting holistic health and wellness.

26. Can encourage emotional release

Somatic therapy can provide a safe space for emotional expression and release, facilitating healing and growth.

27. Can facilitate trauma resolution

By addressing trauma held in the body, somatic therapy can support the resolution of past traumatic experiences.

28. Can support self-expression

Somatic therapy can also encourage authentic self-expression and communication, fostering personal growth.

29. Can increase resilience to stress

Somatic therapy can equip us with tools to cope with stressors effectively, enhancing our resilience.

30. And finally: can enhance our overall quality of life

Through its holistic approach, somatic therapy can improve various aspects of life, leading to a higher overall quality of life.

To me these don't seem like bad things to have, and that's why I'm always pro every healing method, at least to try. Everything will not suit everybody, but unless we give it a try, we won't know.

PART III

"Ask yourself what is important to you, and then have the courage to build your life around your answer."

— Unknown

So here we are, my dear.

It's time. I won't keep you any longer, let's (finally!) jump in!

In This Section You'll Get

    Preparation instructions for your somatic therapy journey

    28-day program overview (plus extra days!)

    Two free days, and understanding how they are important

    Exercises for only 10–15 minutes a day

    Instructions for each day's somatic experiencing exercise

    Pictures to showcase the instructions

    Journaling prompts to help you understand your journey

    Alternative and bonus exercises for you to choose from

    An understanding of how to help yourself

PREPARATION FOR SOMATIC THERAPY

Please, my dear, promise me you'll remember to always create yourself a safe space when doing somatic exercises. Or, actually, any exercises, for that matter! That is super important. Put your devices away, and make sure no-one disturbs you. Tell your close ones you need your own time. (I know it might sometimes be difficult, especially with small children, but they'll learn to respect your space when you guide them.)

You can also with small things make your therapeutic space comfortable and supporting to your therapy exercises. You can make sure the space is somewhat organized (sitting on a lego when meditating can… well, be a little disturbing). If possible, bring a plant in the space, organize pillows or a yoga mat to make a soothing space.

Also, trust your inner guidance. If you feel music will help you, play music. (If you do, I recommend soothing, not too energizing).

The space doesn't have to be a yoga studio, believe me. I have learned to meditate on those Legos and with noises ("Mommy, Mommy, what are you doing there?"), and you will too, if needed. In that case, try to be able to lock the door.

The intention is most important.

I recommend you to always sit a moment before you start, and just ground yourself gently. Concentrate on your breath.

SETTING HEALTHY BOUNDARIES

Learn to listen to yourself and your emotional and bodily messages, my dear. While on your somatic therapy journey, please respect your own healthy boundaries.

These things might guide and help you with your boundaries:

1. **Self-awareness**
   Begin by cultivating an awareness of your bodily sensations, emotions, and triggers. Notice how your body responds to different situations and interactions.

2. **Identify boundaries**

Reflect on areas where you need to establish boundaries to protect your wellbeing. This could include physical boundaries, such as personal space, as well as emotional boundaries, like saying no to tasks that overwhelm you. If any of this book's exercises feels like too much, you can absolutely pass it.

3. **Communicate and/or journal assertively**

Practice expressing your boundaries clearly and assertively. Use "I" statements to communicate your needs and limits without blaming or shaming others. You can journal these thoughts; they can be invaluable later for you to explore.

4. **Listen to your body's wisdom**

Pay attention to physical sensations that signal discomfort or violation of boundaries. Think beforehand or during the exercise what you will and will not try and feel safe to quit at any moment.

EMOTIONAL SAFETY AND SELF-COMPASSION

Your emotional safety is the most important thing in somatic therapy, like any other therapy, and that's why I wanted to list some simple instructions for your emotional safety and self-compassion in your somatic therapy journey. In a way, this book is about your emotional safety and self-compassion, my dear.

Trust your inner knowing. And please, most importantly, in any situation, be kind to yourself.

- Begin by creating a safe and comfortable environment for yourself, free from distractions.
- Practice mindfulness by focusing on your breath and bodily sensations, grounding yourself in the present moment. (You'll

find deeper grounding instructions later.)

- Cultivate self-compassion by acknowledging and accepting your feelings without judgment. (And again, please be kind to yourself!)
- Offer yourself words of kindness and understanding, reminding yourself that it's okay to feel what you're feeling.
- Practice emotional regulation techniques such as deep breathing or progressive muscle relaxation to manage possible overwhelming emotions.
- Set boundaries to protect your emotional wellbeing, both during somatic therapy—and in your daily life. Boundaries are self-love; they tell you and others what's ok and what's not.

It's not just "for fun", emotional safety and self-compassion actually have some deeply rooted benefits:

- **Improved Emotional Regulation**

   Self-compassion and emotional safety techniques help you regulate difficult emotions, reducing the risk of feeling overwhelmed.

- **Enhanced Resilience**

   By cultivating self-compassion, you build resilience to cope with challenging experiences and setbacks.

- **Greater Self-Acceptance**

   Practicing self-compassion fosters greater self-acceptance, allowing you to embrace yourself with kindness and understanding.

- **Deeper Healing**

   Emotional safety creates a nurturing environment where you

can explore and process traumatic experiences, facilitating deeper healing.

- **Increased Self-Awareness**

  By prioritizing emotional safety and self-compassion, you become more aware of your inner experiences and needs, leading to greater self-understanding and growth.

Incorporating self-compassion and emotional safety practices into somatic therapy enhances emotional regulation, resilience, self-acceptance, healing, and self-awareness.

If you remember nothing else, please remember to be kind to yourself.

A BRIEF OVERVIEW OF THE 30-DAY SOMATIC THERAPY PROGRAM

"Trauma is a fact of life. It does not, however, have to be a life sentence."
—Peter A. Levine, Ph.D.

Here, my dear, you can see the layout of our 30-day healing program. Please take a look and let yourself get familiar with it. Pay attention to how you feel about it. What thoughts and feelings arise? You might want to keep journaling alongside of your journey. It may help crystallize your thoughts and feelings, and it may be a precious tool for you later in your journey.

Each chapter of the 30-day program introduces you to the somatic therapy and your journey a little deeper. Our goal is to do it gently and lovingly and support you on every step.

I wanted to design this program to make it as easy as possible for you to fit it in your everyday life. With only about 15 minutes a day you can do the daily exercises. But I also wanted to give you more tools than just the basic 30-day program ones, in case you want to dive deeper, or continue the program later, so I added extra tools for every day, plus journaling questions to help you reflect your feelings, if you do want to journal. (I highly, highly recommend journaling, my dear. Writing is on its own a nice mindful practice, and it also helps you to reflect your journey as a whole path. It can give you so many valuable insights and empowerment, and if there is something I want you to have as takeaways from this book, it's deep insights, healing, and empowerment!)

So please, when you are on your journey, take what you feel resonates with you and leave the rest. You can always get back to the program later, if you feel like it.

WITH ONLY A FEW MINUTES PER DAY YOU CAN FIND SO MANY BEAUTIFUL BENEFITS:

- Deeper mind-body connection
- Deep healing
- Better body awareness
- More loving and nurturing relationship with your body
- Learn to understand your triggers
- Sooth the intensity and frequency of your triggers

DAY 1-5: INTRODUCTION TO SOMATIC AWARENESS

Day 1: Introduction to somatic therapy and trauma healing principles.

Day 2-3: Practice body scanning meditation to increase awareness of bodily sensations.

Day 4: Explore gentle stretching movements to release tension.

Day 5: Reflect on your emotional state during the exercises and journal your observations.

DAY 6-10: BODY-CENTERED MINDFULNESS

Day 6-7: Engage in mindful walking, paying attention to each step and sensation.

Day 8: Try progressive muscle relaxation to release muscular tension.

Day 9: Experiment with mindful eating, savoring each bite, and noticing how your body responds.

Day 10: Become aware of our triggers and learn to cope with them.

DAY 11-15: MOVEMENT AND EXPRESSION

Day 11: Incorporate dance or free-form movement to express emotions non-verbally.

Day 12-13: Explore somatic yoga or tai chi to cultivate balance and flexibility.

Day 14: Engage in creative expression through art, music, or writing.

Day 15: Reflect on any shifts in your body awareness and emotional state.

DAY 16-20: SELF-COMPASSION AND ACCEPTANCE

Day 16: Practice self-compassion meditation, offering kindness to yourself.

Day 17-18: Cultivate gratitude by focusing on the sensations of appreciation in your body.

Day 19: Explore any areas of resistance or discomfort with gentle curiosity.

Day 20: Embrace acceptance of your body and emotions as they are in the present moment.

DAY 21-25: CONNECTION AND SUPPORT

Day 21: Reach out to a trusted friend or therapist to share your somatic therapy journey.

Day 22-23: Engage in a somatic therapy group session or workshop for community support.

Day 24: Practice active listening and empathetic communication with others.

Day 25: Reflect on the role of social connection in supporting somatic healing.

DAY 26-30: INTEGRATION AND MOVING FORWARD

Day 26: Create a somatic self-care plan for continued practice beyond the program.

Day 27-28: Review key somatic techniques and exercises that resonated with you.

Day 29: Set intentions for how you will continue to prioritize somatic awareness in your daily life.

Day 30: Celebrate your journey and acknowledge your growth in somatic awareness and emotional wellbeing.

THE PROGRAM

"People have always understood intuitively that mind and body are not separate."
—Gabor Maté, M. D., from *When The Body Says No*

Welcome to the program, my dear.

I designed this program knowing you might have your daily stressors, and especially I designed this program keeping in mind you might have limited time for this. We have kids to take to and from hobbies, we have stews on the stovetop, and we have meetings and our everyday lives.

I designed this program with the idea of working 15 minutes a day for 30 days and then see how much you have transformed. I also designed a lot of extras just for you to have the choice to take what speaks to you and leave the rest. I wanted you to be able to find your way as easily as possible, with all the support and care you need.

This is the area where momentarily you might not like me so much. But bear with me through this. Sometimes facing our discomfort can be very beneficial for our wellbeing.

Just remember to listen to your inner voice. If something feels uncomfortable, take a moment. Go for a walk, take a day or two and reflect on how you feel.

My therapist used to say, the more uncomfortable something feels, the more important it is to take a closer look, and the more rewarding the outcome can be.

If something really feels overwhelming, trust your inner knowing. Please, seek support if you feel you could use it. There are plenty of trained professionals who would love to help you.

Please remember not to force anything.

LOVING OR AT LEAST EMBRACING THE UNCOMFORTABLE

We know facing our traumas can be... well, uncomfortable. Even scary. It requires us to confront the fears within, to grapple with uncertainty and vulnerability. (This all is also called... well, *human*.) Yet, it is precisely within this discomfort that the seeds of true healing can happen.

Acknowledging our fears is an act of self-compassion, recognizing that, like everyone else, we carry our share of anxieties and uncertainties. It's okay to feel uneasy when peering into the unknown. However, it's important to understand that within this discomfort indeed lies the key to liberation.

So, too, if you are facing discomfort: you are not alone. It is a courageous journey, and with each step, you carve out room for growth, resilience, and a truer, more profound sense of positivity. Embrace the discomfort, and know this: on the other side of that, you may find a more authentic and empowered self.

This is what it's like to be a *real* superhero.

And yes, that is why we added more tools at the end of this book, too.

But please, please remember to center yourself. Always try to work from the place of peace.

PREPARATION FOR SOMATIC EXERCISES

This might be the most single important preparation: Always try to work from a place of peace.

Somatic therapy, and any kind of healing, takes a lot of courage, so please remember, you can already appraise yourself as a superhero. But one thing in our self-healing journey is so important, I wanted to dedicate a whole page to it.

Always, always, always try to work from a state of peace. Sometimes healing can be confusing and messy, and it helps if we do the work from a centered, neutral, peaceful mindset.

And, how to calm and clear ourselves and get to our beautiful center?

Breathe. Gently observe your breathing. You don't have to do anything else, my dear.

Breathe some more.

Set your intention. Sit down and breathe. Close your eyes. Feel the peace settling in.

Meditate. (I've been meditating over 25 years, when it was considered socially on the weird side, and I can tell you *in its simplest form it can be just breathing and gently observing the breathing*. It doesn't have to be anything more complicated than that. You don't have to move to the Himalayas.)

Also, remember to be compassionate towards yourself. Healing can sometimes be messy and confusing, so please, always remember to treat yourself with love.

DAY 1-5: INTRODUCTION TO SOMATIC AWARENESS

In this section we get familiar with the most fundamental somatic therapy tools, giving you an overview and understanding of how to use them in your everyday life.

DAY 1: INTRODUCTION TO SOMATIC THERAPY AND TRAUMA HEALING PRINCIPLES

Please read about the theory in previous pages to understand how somatic therapy works and how it aims to help and support you on your healing journey.

Begin with deep breathing exercises to connect with your body.

Please, also reflect your personal reasons for exploring somatic therapy. Explore, what was it that invited you to read this book? Set intentions for the program and journal about your current state.

Rooting exercises offer numerous benefits, including not only improved stability, balance, and strength but also mental wellbeing. How does it sound to you, my dear? Incorporating these exercises into your daily routine can really enhance your physical performance and promote overall health and wellness.

Consider journaling.

Bonus!

Here you can see a few extra examples of how to explore and strengthen your mind-body connection.

1. **Rocking** (On the ground or in a chair, my dear, in case you thought something else!)

   Do you remember swinging from your childhood? Do you remember how fun it always was? I loved it, and I still do, and luckily I have kids to go to the parks with. They provide a perfect alibi for me, because no-one wants to be viewed as a weirdo.

   If swinging is too out there, you can also just sit on a rocking chair, or even on a sofa or just the floor, and see how the rocking feels.

   Sit comfortably, slowly rock yourself back and forth, and really experience how it feels. Explore the rhythm; let yourself really feel it.

   A Few Benefits of Rocking (Besides It's So Soothing!)

   Regulation of the Nervous System

   Rocking activates the parasympathetic nervous system, promoting relaxation and reducing stress. (Ah, finally a scientific explanation to offer in case someone asks! What a relief!) This regulation of the nervous system can be crucial in somatic therapy for managing trauma and anxiety.

   Release of Tension and Stress

   Rocking promotes the release of tension and stress from the body, providing relief from physical discomfort and emotional distress.

Enhanced Mind-Body Connection

Rocking fosters a connection between physical movement and emotional regulation, emphasizing the mind-body connection central to somatic therapy.

Facilitation of Healing

By inducing a state of relaxation and safety, rocking supports the body's natural healing processes, aiding in the resolution of trauma and emotional wounds.

In summary, rocking can serve as a therapeutic tool in somatic therapy by promoting relaxation, regulating the nervous system, enhancing the mind-body connection, and facilitating the release of tension and stress. Besides, have you done it lately? Isn't it so nurturing and soothing to the soul?

2. Connecting with Nature

Do you remember how the forest smells right after it has rained? Do you remember how freshly cut grass feels under your feet? How do the birds sound just before a storm?

Select a natural environment that feels safe and inviting to you. This could be a forest, beach, park, or any outdoor space with greenery and natural elements.

Engage your senses fully by noticing the sights, sounds, smells, textures, and even tastes of the surrounding environment. Breathe and enjoy. Let your heart rate go down (natural settings tend to do it... should I say naturally.) Use nature's rhythm to guide your breath. Take slow, deep breaths, syncing your inhalations and exhalations with the natural movements around you, such as the swaying of trees or the sound of waves.

Notice how your emotional state shifts in response to the

natural environment, and allow yourself to experience any feelings that arise without judgment.

A Few Benefits of Connecting with Nature

Regulation of the Nervous System

Being in nature can regulate the nervous system in the most beautiful and natural ways, promoting relaxation and reducing stress, which is essential for somatic therapy.

Embodied Experience

Nature facilitates an embodied experience, allowing individuals to connect with their bodies and sensations more deeply, which aligns with the principles of somatic therapy.

Mind-Body Connection

Connecting with nature strengthens the mind-body connection, helping individuals become more aware of how their environment influences their emotions and physical sensations.

Healing Environment

Natural environments offer a healing atmosphere, promoting feelings of safety and relaxation, which are conducive to somatic therapy practices.

Enhanced Emotional Wellbeing

Spending time in nature has been linked to improved mood and emotional wellbeing, which complements the emotional healing goals of somatic therapy.

A SIMPLE ROOTING EXERCISE

Being present in this *present moment* means noticing what's going on–right here, right now.

Just sit and relax for a few minutes. Be present with your breathing. Then use your senses: your eyes, nose, mouth, ears, and body and pay attention. Just observe with loving attention what is going on right here, right now

You can use these sentences to help you. You can even journal, if you like.

I can see…
I can smell…
I can taste…
I can hear…

Journaling prompts to help you reflect:

What was it that invited you to read this book?

How do you feel now?

What are your intentions for your somatic therapy journey?

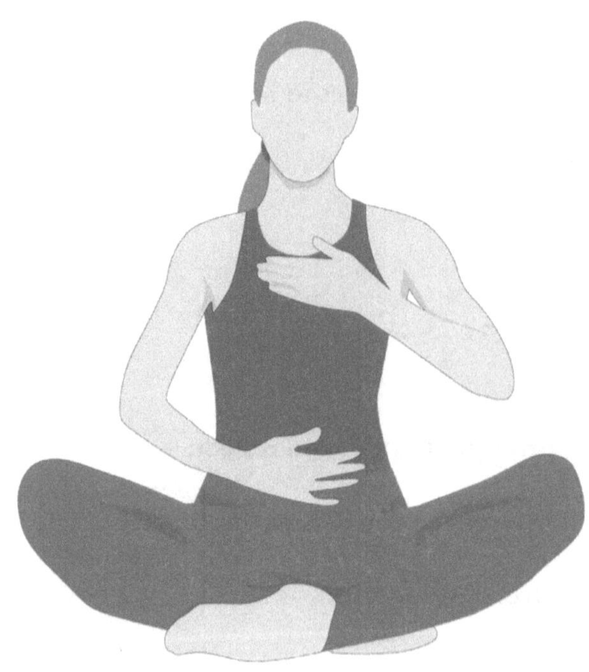

Figure 1 Breathing is one of the most amazing tools we have, and we carry it around with us… all times!

DAY 2: THE BEAUTY OF OUR BREATHING

We have this beautiful tool with us *our whole lives*, from the beginning to the very end. It's called breathing.

We in the Western world have not quite understood how incredibly powerful a tool our breathing actually is. In the East they have known this for thousands of years. (Also, possibly, we had that wisdom, too, before we got too carried away with industrialization, a concept called time, and smartphones).

Just in recent years our science has woken up to actually explore it a bit, and breathing has become one of The Things, for example for top athletes and performers of our whole lovely planet. (Yes, it's *that* powerful. I'm not joking.)

It is so powerful, breath work—especially box breathing—is being taught to NAVY Seals (Divine, 2016). Do you think they'd use it in high stress situations if it wasn't effective?

No wonder they have had the *pranayama* practices for thousands of years.

DIAPHRAGMATIC BREATHING

Please understand, when we talk about breathwork, we mean deep breathing.

(We don't mean the shallow breathing that usually takes place when we see a lion behind the bush or get an email from our boss.)

(And yes, the previous examples can very much trigger the same reaction in our bodies, my dear.)

The deep breathing technique can also be called diaphragmatic breathing, also beautifully known as belly breathing, which involves engaging our diaphragm, a large muscle located beneath our lungs, to really help gain relaxation and effective oxygen exchange.

Diaphragmatic breathing entails inhaling deeply through our nose, really allowing the abdomen to expaaaaaaand as the diaphragm contracts downward. Exhalation occurs slowly through pursed lips, with the abdomen deflating as the diaphragm relaaaaaaaaaaxes.

THE SCIENCE OF HOW BREATHWORK AFFECTS OUR EMOTIONAL REGULATION AND STRESS REDUCTION

1. **Physiological Effects**

   Deep breathing techniques, such as breathwork, stimulate the parasympathetic nervous system, triggering the relaxation response. This can lead to decreased heart rate, blood pressure, and cortisol levels, promoting a sense of calmness.

2. **Emotional Regulation**

   Breathwork enhances emotional regulation by influencing brain regions involved in emotional processing, such as the amygdala and prefrontal cortex. It increases activity in the prefrontal cortex, responsible for executive function and decision-making, while reducing amygdala activity linked to fear and stress responses.

3. **Respiratory Sinus Arrhythmia (RSA)**

   Breathwork can modulate RSA, the natural variation in heart rate during the breathing cycle. Increased RSA correlates with better emotion regulation, improved attention, and reduced stress. Breathwork techniques like coherent breathing synchronize RSA with respiration, fostering emotional stability.

4. **And of Course, the Mind-Body Connection**

Breathwork can foster mindfulness by anchoring attention to the present moment through an awareness of breath. This mindfulness practice enhances self-awareness, emotional clarity, and resilience, enabling individuals to respond more effectively to stressors.

5. **Neuroplasticity**

Regular breathwork can induce beautiful neuroplastic changes in our brain, promoting long-term emotional regulation and stress resilience. It can enhance neural connectivity and neurogenesis in brain regions associated with emotion regulation, leading to sustained improvements in mental wellbeing.

In summary, breathwork positively influences both physiological and psychological mechanisms, contributing to enhanced emotional regulation and stress reduction.

(By the way. James Nestor writes in his beautiful book *Breath—The New Science of a Lost Art,* which I would recommend everyone to read, not only once, but several times, most of the ancient (religious) ritual humming is based on the incredible power of our breathing. They knew the power of regulating our mind and body with our breathing already *then*, and we are slowly re-learning it, thank goodness.)

If you would only like to hear *one* advice for breathing, according to many articles, try to breathe *less*. Fewer breaths, and less air.

But if you are like most of us, you would like to know more and have more exercises. Here you are, my dear.

A FEW BREATHING EXERCISES

Always aim for diaphragmatic breathing, which means deep, calm breathing. Like this:

- Inhale slooooooowly through your nose. Allow your diaphragm to expand.
- Exhale slooooooooowly through your mouth. Feel your belly contract.
- With each breath, let your consciousness rest on the rise and fall of your abdomen.

BOX BREATHING

1. **Find a Comfortable Position**

   Sit or lie down in a comfortable position. You can close your eyes if it helps you relax.

2. **Focus on Your Breath**

   Begin by taking a slow, deep breath in through your nose. Feel your abdomen expand as you fill your lungs with air.

3. **Hold Your Breath**

   Once you've inhaled fully, hold your breath for a count of four seconds. Maintain a steady and relaxed posture during this pause.

4. **Exhale Slowly**

   Slowly exhale through your mouth for a count of four seconds. Focus on completely emptying your lungs as you release the breath.

5. **Hold Your Breath Again**

After exhaling, hold your breath for another count of four seconds. Keep your body relaxed and tension-free during this pause.

6. **Repeat**

Continue the cycle by inhaling deeply through your nose for four seconds, holding for four seconds, exhaling slowly through your mouth for four seconds, and holding again for four seconds.

7. **Practice Regularly**

Aim to practice box breathing for several minutes, gradually increasing the duration as you become more comfortable with the technique.

8. **Stay Relaxed**

Throughout the exercise, try to maintain a relaxed and calm demeanor. Focus on the rhythm of your breath and allow yourself to let go of any tension or stress.

You can do box breathing anywhere and anytime you need to relax or reduce stress.

4-7-8 Breathing

1. **Origins**

The 4-7-8 breathing technique originated from pranayama, an ancient yogic practice that focuses on breath control. This technique also aims to promote relaxation and ease stress.

2. **Technique:**

- Begin by sitting or lying down in a comfortable position.
- Close your eyes and take a deep breath in through your nose

for a count of four seconds.

- Hold your breath for seven seconds.
- Slowly exhale through your mouth for eight seconds, making a whooshing sound.
- Repeat the cycle for a total of four breaths or as desired.

3. **Science** Behind 4-7-8 Breathing

- The 4-7-8 breathing technique is believed to activate the body's relaxation response by stimulating the parasympathetic nervous system. This promotes a sense of calmness and reduces stress. Deep breathing exercises like 4-7-8 breathing can increase oxygen intake, improve lung function, and lower blood pressure. It also can help regulate the autonomic nervous system, leading to a reduction in anxiety and improved emotional wellbeing.

4. **Practice:**

- Practice 4-7-8 breathing regularly, whenever you feel stressed or anxious.
- Over time, consistent practice can enhance its effectiveness in promoting relaxation and overall wellbeing.

By incorporating 4-7-8 breathing into your routine, you can harness its calming effects to manage stress and cultivate a greater sense of peace and tranquility.

JOURNALING PROMPTS TO GUIDE YOU TO UNDERSTAND YOUR BREATHING BETTER:

When was the last time you paid attention to your breath?

How did the breathing exercise feel?

Do you have any thoughts on how breathing exercises will help you?

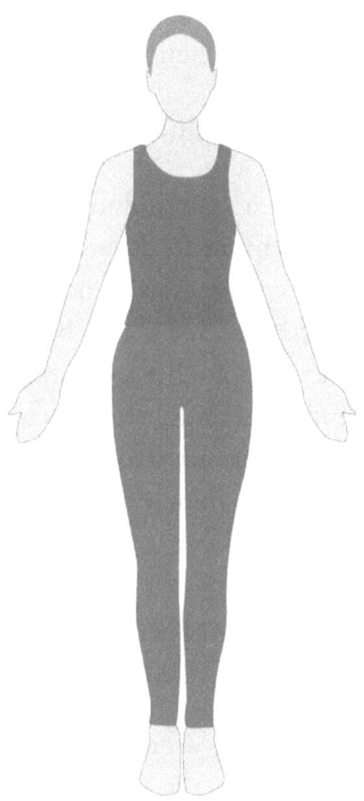

Figure 2: Body scanning and breathing remarkable benefits in the realm of somatic therapy.

DAY 3: BODY SCANNING MEDITATION TO INCREASE AWARENESS OF BODILY SENSATIONS

Body Scan Meditation

Welcome to the transformative journey of body scan meditation, a profound practice deeply rooted in somatic therapy. In this introductory chapter, we delve into the essence of body scanning meditation and its remarkable benefits in the realm of somatic therapy.

Understanding Body Scan Meditation

Body scan meditation is a mindfulness technique that involves systematically directing attention to different parts of our body, from head to toe, with focused awareness and non-judgmental observation. (If you remember nothing else from this book, remember the word non-judgmental, and please apply that to yourself and others!) Through body scanning and gentle guidance, we can cultivate a deep sense of presence and connection with our physical sensations, emotions, and inner experiences. The famous mind-body connection!

BENEFITS OF BODY SCAN MEDITATION IN SOMATIC THERAPY

1. **Enhanced Somatic Awareness**

   Body scanning meditation fosters heightened awareness of bodily sensations, facilitating a deeper understanding of the mind-body connection.

2. **Calming the Nervous System**

   By promoting relaxation and reducing stress, body scan meditation helps us to calm the nervous system, offering relief from anxiety and tension. I don't know about you, but to me it's very welcome!

3. **Trauma Healing**

    In somatic therapy, body scanning meditation serves as a powerful tool for trauma healing, allowing us to safely explore and release stored trauma held within our body.

4. **Pain Management**

    Body scan meditation can aid in pain management by promoting relaxation and shifting focus away from discomfort, offering — again! — a holistic approach to pain relief.

5. **Mind-Body Integration**

    Through regular practice, body scan meditation facilitates greater integration of mind and body, fostering holistic wellbeing and emotional resilience.

So, let's explore the body scanning.

1. **Introduction**
    Find a comfortable position, either lying down or sitting with your back straight. Close your eyes gently and take a few deep breaths to center yourself.

2. **Grounding**: Begin by bringing your awareness to the contact points between your body and the surface beneath you. Feel the support beneath you, grounding you to the present moment.

3. **Starting Point**: Direct your attention to your toes. Notice any sensations in your toes, such as warmth, tingling, or pressure. Allow your breath to flow naturally as you focus on your toes for a few moments.

4. **Progression**: Slowly move your attention up through your feet, ankles, calves, and thighs, scanning each part of your body with curiosity and openness. Notice any areas of tension or

relaxation without trying to change anything.

5. **Abdomen and Chest**: Shift your attention to your abdomen and chest. Notice the rise and fall of your breath as you observe the sensations in this area. Allow any feelings or emotions to arise and pass without judgment.

6. **Shoulders and Arms**: Bring your awareness to your shoulders, arms, and hands. Notice any sensations of heaviness or lightness, tension, or ease. Allow your shoulders to soften as you breathe deeply.

7. **Neck and Head**: Finally, scan your neck, face, and head. Notice any areas of tightness or relaxation. Soften the muscles of your face and jaw as you continue to breathe deeply.

8. **Whole Body Awareness**: Take a moment to expand your awareness to your entire body. Feel the interconnectedness of your body as a whole, grounded, and present in this moment.

9. **Closing**: When you're ready, gently bring your attention back to your breath. Take a few more deep breaths, and slowly begin to wiggle your fingers and toes. When you feel ready, open your eyes.

This body scan meditation can help you cultivate greater awareness of your body, reduce stress, and promote relaxation.

You are welcome to record yourself (or a friend) narrating the body-scanning meditation and listen to it whenever you have the need. I'll add another, longer body-scan meditation for you in the bonus chapter, if this is "your meditation." (As with everything, we have preferences in meditations, and body-scanning can be incredibly healing for some people. If you are one of those people, you might want to try the longer script as well.)

And again, my dear, consider journaling.

Journaling prompts to help you:

How did the body scan feel?

Was there anything specific you noticed? Any body parts?

Did the body scan connect your mind and body?

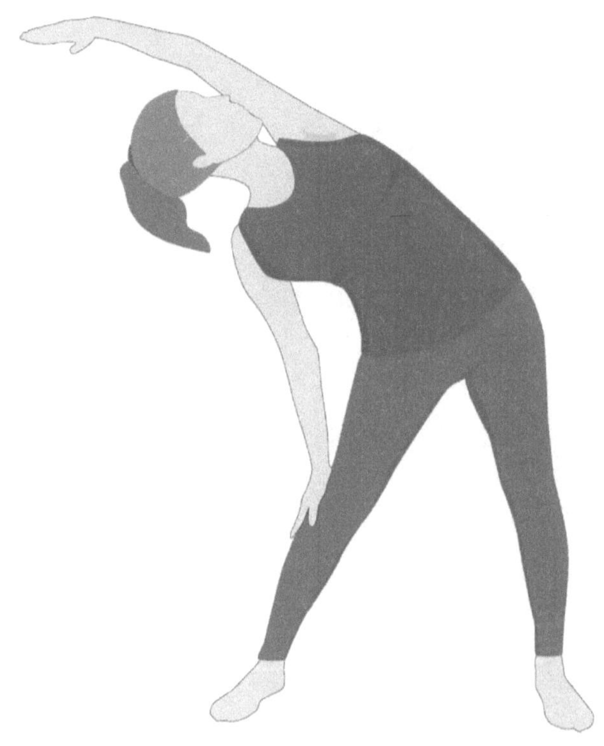

Figure 3 Listen to your body, breath deep and slow. Remember, it's not a race!

DAY 4: EXPLORE GENTLE STRETCHING MOVEMENTS TO RELEASE TENSION

In the fast-paced rhythm of our modern lives, stress and tension often accumulate in our bodies, manifesting as tightness and discomfort. Amidst this hustle and bustle, finding moments of relaxation and rejuvenation becomes essential for our overall wellbeing. Gentle stretching movements offer a simple yet powerful way to release tension, restore balance, and nurture the body-mind connection.

1. **Understanding the Importance of Movement**

   Our bodies are designed for movement, yet sedentary lifestyles and prolonged periods of sitting can lead to muscle stiffness and decreased flexibility. Incorporating gentle stretching into our daily routine promotes circulation, enhances joint mobility, and revitalizes our physical vitality.

2. **Embracing Mindful Awareness**

   Engaging in stretching movements provides an opportunity to cultivate a mindful awareness of our body's sensations and needs. By tuning into the present moment and listening to the messages of our body, we develop a deeper understanding of our physical state and foster a sense of self-care and compassion.

3. **Releasing Physical and Emotional Tension**

   Tension held in the body often reflects underlying emotional stressors. Through gentle stretching, we create space for the release of both physical and emotional tension, allowing blocked energy to flow freely and promoting a sense of ease and relaxation.

4. **Fostering Connection and Relaxation**

Stretching movements invite us to reconnect with our bodies and acknowledge the inherent wisdom within. As we move through gentle stretches with intention and mindfulness, we cultivate a sense of relaxation and inner peace, fostering a harmonious relationship between body, mind, and spirit.

5. **Embarking on a Journey of Self-Exploration**

Exploring gentle stretching movements is not only about physical flexibility but also about embarking on a journey of our self-exploration and self-discovery. Each stretch becomes an opportunity to deepen our connection with ourselves, honor our bodies, and embrace the present moment with openness and acceptance.

Join us on a journey to explore the transformative power of gentle stretching movements as we step on a path of relaxation, rejuvenation, and holistic wellbeing.

DAY 5: REFLECT ON YOUR EMOTIONAL STATE DURING THE EXERCISES AND JOURNAL YOUR OBSERVATIONS

Again, the journaling, my dear.

Journaling prompts to help you:

Describe how your body feels before and after engaging in a gentle stretching routine.

Reflect on any tension or stress you noticed in your body during the stretching session and explore its possible sources.

Write about any emotions that arose during the stretching movements and how they affected your overall mood.

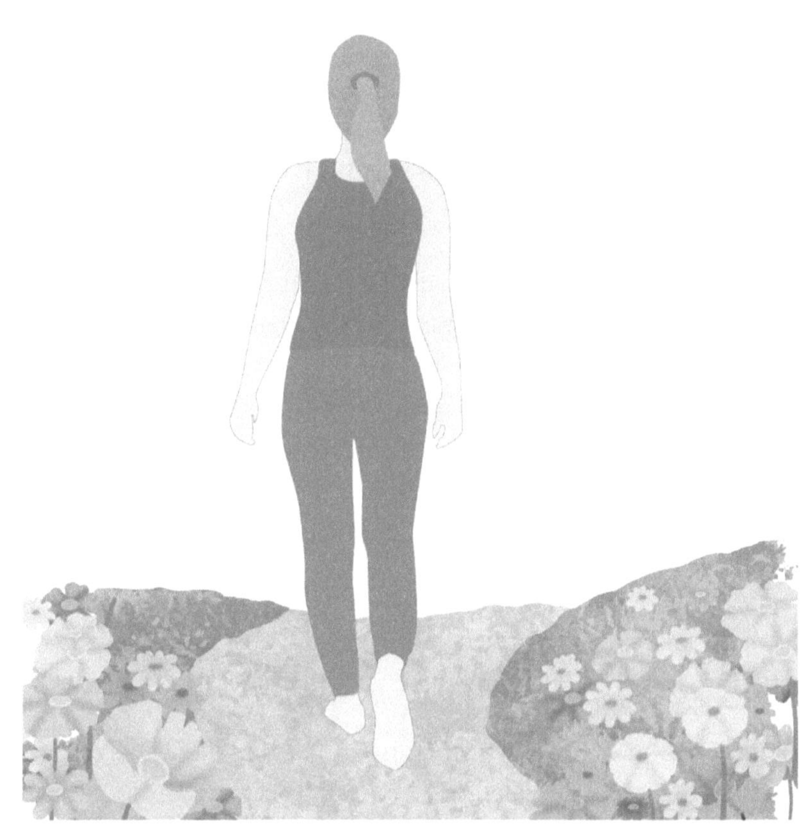

Figure 4 I love barefoot walking, and I would do it year-round if the winters weren't cold here. Read the beautiful benefits of going barefoot!

DAY 6-10: BODY-CENTERED MINDFULNESS

Day 6-7: Engage In Mindful Walking, Paying Attention To Each Step

Mindful walking, a practice rooted in mindfulness, holds profound benefits within our realm of somatic therapy. This intentional form of movement combines the principles of mindfulness with the physical act of walking, fostering a holistic approach to healing and wellbeing. Mindful walking can help you enhance your **somatic awareness, emotional regulation and grounding and centering yourself, among other things.**

Mindful walking in nature actually has a solid scientific background in trauma healing. For example, the U.S. Navy has scientifically researched surfing and hiking as a therapy form for MDD (major depressive disorder) and PTSD (Post Traumatic Stress Disorder). PTSD can cause depression, sleeping problems, tension, and anger. These all can lead to violence, addictions, and other severe problems. This research was published in 2019. In short, the idea of the U.S. Navy research was to engage therapy with the *natural environment outdoors and physical activity*.

If it works for Navy Seals and very severe trauma reactions, I'm pretty sure it works for others, too.

Since I am a wellbeing science nerd, I would like to share this with you, too, to slightly deepen the topic and back it up with neuroscience.

Neuroscientist Dr. Andrew Huberman has spoken about optic flow and its affects on our nervous system; for example, in the RichRoll podcast. He talks about how taking a walk where you just let your mind go, is very powerful—and so is optic flow.

"Self-generated optic flow by walking, running, or cycling, shifts the brain into a state of relaxation," he says.

Relaxation, which is not seeing in a stationary state.

He goes on to say, "When you move through space, you're active, there's a natural calming of the neuro circuits involved in threat and threat detection."

He continues this being the basis of EMDR (Eye Movement Desensitization Reprocessing), a trauma-treatment method. The lateralized eye movements lower stress by quieting the activity in the amygdala, the limbic structure in the brain, that's primarily responsible for threat detection and stress.

Huberman further presents a therapist called Francine Shapiro first having observed her problems didn't seem to be so bad when she was walking, and that might be useful to others too.

(Well, yes!)

I could go on forever about the brain science of this, but since we only have one book and a lot of topics, I'll have to continue.

But please remember, don't go do EMDR therapy on your own, since in my opinion it requires a professional practitioner to help, but as a takeaway please remember: walks, runs, and cycling promotes healing also from the neuroscience point of view.

1. **Mindful walk**

    Mindful walking exercises emphasize paying attention to the sensations in your feet as they make contact with the ground. This cultivates mindfulness, improves balance, and fosters a sense of connection with the earth. Don't stress over it. Just let yourself just experience how it feels.

2. **Barefoot walking**

    I have always loved barefoot walking, even as an adult. Below are some of the benefits.

3. **Sensory Awareness**

    Barefoot walking stimulates the senses, allowing individuals to become more aware of their body's sensations and movements. This heightened sensory awareness is fundamental to somatic therapy, which really emphasizes the mind-body connection.

4. Grounding and Mindfulness

Walking barefoot literally connects you with the earth, promoting a sense of grounding and mindfulness. This practice encourages present-moment awareness, which is one of the key aspects of somatic therapy.

6. Stress Reduction

Barefoot walking in natural environments, such as grass or sand, has been shown to reduce stress and anxiety levels. This aligns with the goals of somatic therapy, which aims to alleviate physical and emotional tension.

5. Enhanced Body Awareness

Also, besides being fun, walking barefoot strengthens the smaller muscles, tendons, and ligaments in the feet in your body, improving proprioception and body awareness. This heightened awareness of bodily sensations supports the somatic therapy process.

JOURNALING PROMPTS TO GUIDE YOU: REFLECT ON THE SENSATIONS IN YOUR BODY AS YOU WALKED MINDFULLY: WHAT DID YOU NOTICE ABOUT YOUR POSTURE, MUSCLE TENSION, AND BREATH?

Explore the connection between your thoughts and bodily sensations: How did your thoughts influence the way you moved and perceived your environment?

Did any emotions arise during your mindful walk? How did walking mindfully (or even barefoot) impact your mood and emotional state?

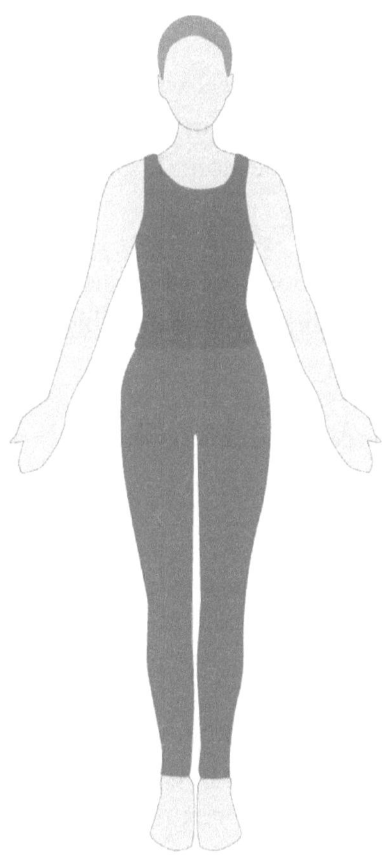

Figure 5 Body scanning is a wonderful way to connect with your body.

DAY 8: FIND EMOTIONS IN YOUR BODY

My therapist was annoyingly calm, as always. She was an older lady, and super laser focused as she sat on her brown armchair.

She asked, "Where do you feel this feeling in your body?"

The first time she asked that, I was staggered. What was she talking about? What body? Hey, lady, I am here talking about the dramas of my life, and she asks a stupid question. (I only thought this, never said this, I swear.)

With time, I learned (note: even I learned, so you can, too, my dear) to explore my feelings and how unbelievably connected they were (and are) in my body.

How did I not understand this before?

I learned, but it was hard.

Then my therapist asked another question.

"*How* does it feel?"

How does it feel? Are you kidding me? I just learned with huge effort, sweating, to even understand my feelings are connected to my body. And now you want to know even more? Is nothing ever enough for you?

Of course, I never said anything. I was a good girl and tried to answer something to her question.

(Good girls never complain, right?!)

A FEW EXERCISES TO HELP YOU LOCATE YOUR FEELINGS IN YOUR BODY

1. Body Mapping

Use a body map or drawing to identify where you feel different emotions in your body. You can note any patterns or recurring sensations associated with specific emotions.

2. Journaling

Write in a journal about your physical sensations and emotions. Reflect on how different emotions manifest in your body and how they impact your overall wellbeing.

3. Body Scan Meditation

Sit or lie down in a comfortable position. Close your eyes and bring your awareness to different parts of your body, starting from your toes and slowly moving up to your head. Notice any sensations or tensions in each area and observe any emotions that arise along with them.

4. Deep Breathing

Practice deep breathing exercises, focusing on the sensations of your breath as it enters and leaves your body. Pay attention to any emotions that surface during this mindful breathing practice.

5. Mindful Movement

Engage in gentle movements such as yoga, tai chi, or qigong, paying close attention to how your body feels with each movement. Notice any areas of tension or relaxation and observe any corresponding emotions.

Prompts to help you reflect and journal:

1. Where in your body do you notice tension or discomfort when you experience stress or anxiety? Describe these sensations and explore any emotions associated with them.

2. Reflect on a challenging situation you encountered today. How did your body respond to this stressor? What emotions did you feel, and where did you feel them in your body?

3. Think about a recent joyful or peaceful moment. What physical sensations did you experience during that time? How did these sensations manifest in different parts of your body?

DAY 9: EXPERIMENT WITH MINDFUL EATING AND SAVORING EACH BITE

I don't remember what exact therapeutic training it was, but I do remember the question exactly. The trainer looked to her audience, us, and took a step forward on the stage. "Who do you shower with?" she said.

We in the audience were absolutely surprised. The keynote speaker continued. "Who do you go to sleep with? Or eat with?"

He asked, when had we been in the moment, without carrying our bosses, co-workers, disagreements at work, our ex-spouses, siblings, parents in our heads, without concentrating on what we were actually doing.

We looked at each other. The keynote speaker was so right.

Who do you shower with? Or eat with?

I would like to give you tools to actually eat with yourself and with the company you are with, and not with your boss or ex-spouse. Starting with mindful eating might be an easy way to get ourselves on our way.

SCIENTIFIC BENEFITS OF MINDFUL EATING

1. **Increased Pleasure When Eating**

Practicing mindfulness while eating can enhance the enjoyment of food and the overall eating experience. It does taste better when eaten slowly rather than just shoveling the food down the throat, right?!

2. **Weight Management**

Mindful eating promotes a renewed sense of hunger and fullness, and it can aid in weight management and maintenance.

3. **Improved Self-esteem**

By fostering self-awareness and acceptance, mindful eating can lead to improved self-esteem.

4. **Empowerment**
Mindful eating empowers us to make conscious choices about our food intake and eating habits, leading to a sense of control over our health.

5. **Reduced Stress**

Mindful eating practices have been associated with stress reduction, contributing to overall wellbeing.

6. **Improved Digestion**

Being present and attentive while eating can aid in better digestion and nutrient absorption. For example, when we chew our food better, the food digests better, and it's free! We don't have to buy expensive digestive supplements.

101

7. **Lowered Risk of Heart Disease**

Mindful eating may reduce the ratio of triglycerides to HDL (good) cholesterol, potentially lowering the risk of heart disease.

8. **Improved Psychological Wellbeing**

Mindful eating has been linked to greater psychological wellbeing, including reduced stress and anxiety.

You might have read about how stress is connected to gut health? Mindful eating and somatic therapy can help you with those.

I was diagnosed with IBS (irritable bowel syndrome) almost 20 years ago, and I would be the first to say, stress does have a direct line to the gut.

JOURNALING PROMPTS ABOUT MINDFUL EATING:

1. What thoughts arise as you took the first bite of your food during the mindful eating exercise?

2. How did these thoughts influence your experience of eating and your bodily sensations?

3. As you chewed your food mindfully, what physical sensations did you notice? How did the act of chewing slowly and intentionally affect your perception of taste and texture?

4. What emotions emerged as you focused on the sensory experience of eating? How did these emotions manifest in your body, and how did your awareness of them evolve throughout the exercise?

DAY 10: UNDERSTANDING YOUR TRIGGERS CAN HELP YOU HEAL

"This has been one of the most important tools in my life," said my colleague, author Claudia Berg.

She told me, "I will share a secret with you. My therapist used to listen to me with a (sometimes annoyingly) calm, loving expression on her face. She sat calmly in her armchair, while I was my usual emotional mess, rambling about this and that with high emotional charge. (Meaning, usually furious about something. Usually around eighty-nine on a scale of one to one hundred.)"

She took a moment and said, "She listened. She never interrupted me. Then, when I (finally!) shut my mouth, she would ask this most annoying question."

I leaned in, even when I almost knew the answer. Berg paused before saying, "She asked, 'What happened **BEFORE** this'?"

She said the question really got to her. "I usually had no idea. Her question annoyed me. Badly."

Berg told me, "But she explained with that question we can get onto something really important, that being *our **emotional triggers.***"

Thank you, Berg, for your honesty—and most of all, the simple explanation of the importance of understanding our triggers.

I wanted to grant you this annoying question too, and remember, sometimes something that annoys the most, can also heal the most. (This was another really annoying thing my therapist used to say.)

So, my dear, welcome to trigger hunting.

Somatic therapy indeed guides us to become aware of when our bodies are telling us we're stressed or triggered. It can be anything from **muscle tension, stomach aches, headaches, shallow breathing,**

too, for example, numbness. Somatic therapy also can help us learn how to calm or discharge that stress, tension, and trauma.

Triggers in somatic therapy are like little alarm clocks for your body, but instead of waking you up, they shake loose past experiences that your body's been holding onto. Picture it: you're cruising along, living your best life, and then bam! Something sets off your internal alarm system, making you feel all sorts of things you thought you'd buried. But fear not! Somatic therapy swoops in like a superhero to help you make sense of these triggers. It's like having a trusty sidekick guiding you through a labyrinth of emotions and sensations, helping you reclaim your power. So, next time a trigger sneaks up on you, embrace it like an unexpected plot twist in your life's story. With somatic therapy by your side, you'll emerge stronger, wiser, and ready to conquer whatever comes your way.

1. Definition

Triggers can be sensory cues, thoughts, emotions, or situations that resemble or symbolize past trauma. These stimuli activate the body's fight-or-flight response, leading to heightened arousal or emotional distress.

2. Impact

Triggers disrupt emotional regulation and may manifest as panic attacks, flashbacks, or physical symptoms, like sweating or trembling. They can hinder daily functioning and quality of life, prompting avoidance behaviors to minimize exposure to triggering stimuli.

3. Treatment

Somatic therapy addresses triggers by integrating body-focused interventions to regulate the nervous system's response. Techniques such as grounding exercises, breathwork, and body awareness help clients manage physiological arousal and regain a sense of safety.

4. Healing

By exploring triggers within the therapeutic relationship, clients develop resilience and coping strategies to navigate triggering experiences. Somatic therapy aims to release stored trauma from the body, fostering emotional processing and integration for long-term healing.

Understanding triggers in somatic therapy empowers us to engage in self-awareness and self-regulation practices, promoting recovery and emotional wellbeing.

Trigger Hunting Tool

When we can recognize our triggers, it can give us enormous emotional freedom. (And I might add: Sometimes the recognizing process can be a bit rough, but you can get through it. Remember, you are not alone. We are with you.)

Write down and explore:

Date/Time

Emotion/Mood (Intensity 1—100)

Thoughts What happened? Where? When? With who? What did you think and feel?

Pay attention **what happened just before the emotion/mood?**

Journaling prompts to help you become aware of your triggers:

1. Reflect on a recent triggering experience. What physical sensations did you notice in your body during the trigger?

2. And, you probably guessed what's coming—the annoying question: what happened before that?

3. Explore the emotions that arose when you were triggered. How did these emotions feel in your body? Were there any specific areas of tension or discomfort? Describe and acknowledge these sensations.

4. Observe how you responded to the trigger. How did your body instinctively react, and were these reactions helpful or hindering? Reflect on any insights gained from observing your responses.

DAY 11-15: MOVEMENT AND EXPRESSION

Movement and expression play vital roles in somatic therapy, offering avenues for us to explore and process our inner experiences beyond the normal verbal communication. (Getting us out of our heads, so to speak.) Through gentle movement exercises, such as mindful breathing, yoga, or simple body movements, individuals can cultivate an awareness of our bodily sensations and emotions.

We can learn to know ourselves better!

Likewise, creative expression techniques, such as drawing, journaling, or guided imagery, can provide beautiful outlets for expressing and integrating emotions stored in our bodies. These approaches can foster a deeper understanding of ourselves, promoting healing and wellbeing by honoring our body's innate wisdom. In somatic therapy, movement and expression serve as gateways to accessing and releasing the hidden pent-up emotions, again, facilitating a holistic journey towards our healing and self-discovery.

DAY 11: CONSIDER INCORPORATING DANCE OR FREE-FORM MOVEMENT TO EXPRESS EMOTIONS NON-VERBALLY

"Dance like nobody is watching!"
—Unknown

Ask yourself: *What if?*

What if you could move freely, without any pressure or stress about how you look? Take a look at small children. They have absolutely no stress, and their movement is free and creative.

1. **Mind-Body Connection**

   Movement can serve as a bridge to integrate our psychological and physiological experiences, promoting holistic healing.

2. **Emotional Regulation**

   Physical movement and expression in somatic therapy facilitate emotional regulation by allowing us to release, again, our pent-up emotions and reduce emotional arousal.

3. **Enhanced Self-Awareness**

   Engaging in movement and expression exercises fosters greater self-awareness, helping us recognize and understand our physical and emotional sensations deeper.

4. **Stress Reduction**

   Movement-based somatic therapies have been associated with stress reduction, as physical activity can help ease tension and promote relaxation.

5. **Trauma Recovery**

Movement-based somatic therapies, such as dance/movement therapy, have been shown to aid in trauma recovery by providing a beautiful non-verbal outlet for expression and processing traumatic experiences.

DAY 12-13: EXPLORE SOMATIC YOGA TO CULTIVATE BALANCE AND FLEXIBILITY

Somatic yoga can empower you to beautifully nurture your wellbeing from the inside out. As we know, we store our emotions and stress within our bodies, and somatic yoga can help us release the tension.

Somatic yoga movements can emphasize conscious embodiment and internal awareness during yoga practice. Unlike traditional yoga, somatic yoga focuses on the sensory experience of each movement, encouraging us to tune into bodily sensations, emotions, and subtle shifts within us. These movements aim to release chronic muscle tension, alleviate stress, and promote holistic wellbeing by engaging the relaxation response in our nervous system.

In somatic therapy, somatic yoga serves as a therapeutic tool to address different physical and emotional concerns. Through gentle, mindful movements, we can explore our body-mind connection, cultivate mindfulness, and enhance proprioception—the awareness of our body in space. Somatic yoga movements often involve slow, fluid sequences, allowing us to reconnect with our bodies and access deeper layers of self-awareness.

By integrating somatic yoga into our healing journey, we can harness its benefits to support trauma recovery, manage chronic pain, reduce anxiety, and foster emotional resilience. Ultimately, somatic yoga movements offer a pathway for us to embody healing, self-discovery, and inner transformation.

Please remember: **Somatic movement should never be painful. If you feel pain, take a break and/or ease the exercise.**

SOME BEAUTIFUL BENEFITS OF SOMATIC YOGA MOVEMENTS:

Release and Healing

Somatic yoga aims to release chronic muscle tension and patterns related possibly to stress, trauma, or even repetitive movements. By addressing these physical imbalances, you can experience both physical and emotional healing.

Neuroplasticity

Our brain is incredible. It has the ability to rewire itself; for example, through repetitive movement and focused attention. Somatic yoga movement can help the rewiring of your brain and nervous system through neural pathways, helping to improve movement patterns and increase body awareness.

A FEW SIMPLE BUT POWERFUL SOMATIC YOGA EXERCISES

Cat-Cow Stretch

Begin on your hands and knees in a tabletop position. Inhale, arching your back and lifting your head and tailbone towards the ceiling (Cow Pose). Exhale, rounding your spine and tucking your chin towards your chest (Cat Pose). Move through these two poses in a flowing motion, syncing your breath with the movement. Repeat for a few rounds.

CAT COW POSE

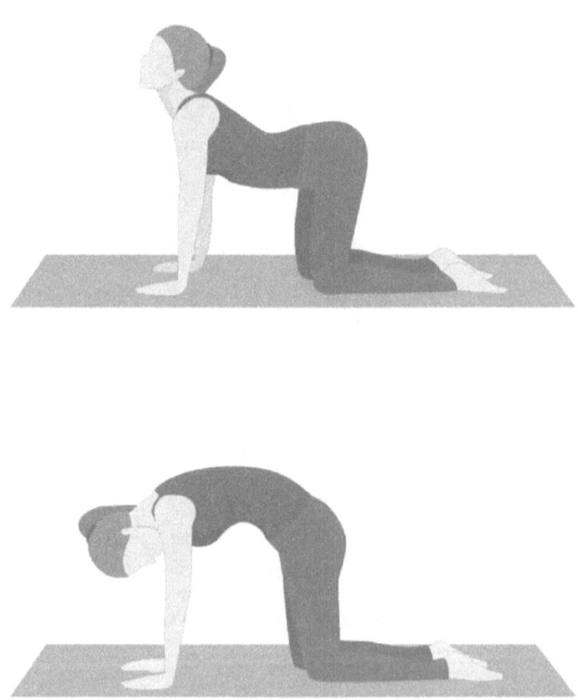

Figure 6 Cat Cow is wonderful for your back. Always listen to your body, start gently. Yoga poses are not a race, or a competition.

Butterfly Stretch

Sit down on the floor or mat with your legs extended in front of you. Bend your knees and bring the soles of your feet together, allowing your knees to fall out to the sides. Hold your feet with your hands, interlacing your fingers around your toes if possible. Keep your back straight and tall, engaging your core muscles.

Gently press your knees down towards the floor with your elbows, feeling a stretch in your inner thighs and groin area. Hold the stretch for 10-30 seconds, breathing deeply and relaxing into the stretch. If you want to deepen the stretch, gently flap your knees up and down, like the wings of a butterfly, while maintaining the pressure downwards. Release the stretch slowly and repeat as needed.

Remember to listen to your body and avoid pushing yourself too far into the stretch. You can gently increase the intensity over time as your flexibility improves.

Gentle Wall Butterfly Pose (Wall Baddha Konasana)

Set Up: Place a folded blanket or mat on the floor near a wall for cushioning.

Lie Down close to the wall and gently swing your legs up onto the wall as you lower your back onto the floor.

Position Your Legs: Bend your knees and bring the soles of your feet together, allowing your knees to open out to the sides to form a diamond shape.

Adjust: Move your hips closer or further from the wall to find a comfortable stretch in your hips and groin.

Relax: Rest your arms by your sides or on your abdomen. Close your eyes and take slow, deep breaths.

Hold the Pose: Stay in this position for 5-10 minutes, focusing on releasing tension and breathing deeply.

Exit the Pose: To come out of the pose, bring your knees together, roll to one side, and gently push yourself up to a seated position.

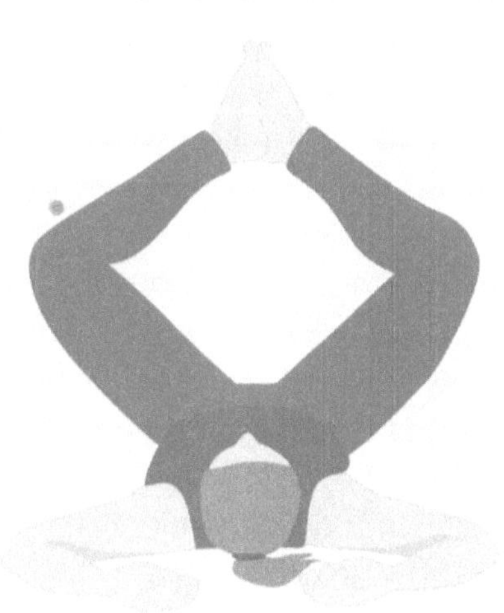

Figure 7 Butterfly comes in many forms, always listen to yourself how to do it. Start easy, and gradually deepen it.

DAY 14: ENGAGE IN CREATIVE EXPRESSION THROUGH ART

I wanted to add this day to you to dedicate just to enjoy art. Any kind of art! Music, dance, writing, pottery, sewing… Or just doing something with your body or mind, or, actually, not just doing something, but… enjoying and letting yourself heal during the rest.

Sometimes I have seen a few days of just enjoying in the middle of healing programs can do wonders. (*Literally* wonders!)

Pauses are crucial in… basically everything. Learning, healing—in life! In somatic therapy, pauses are sometimes good.

Today, you can just enjoy and rest with the little moments of beauties in your life. You can journal, if you like, explore your feelings and how this day made you feel on your healing journey, but you don't have to.

Just remember, you are not alone. You are not crazy. We are here with you, every step on your way.

Why is a rest day so important in healing?

There are many reasons, my dear. Not only to get some air, but the neuroscience backs it up, too.

1. **Neural Integration**

    Rest days allow our brain to process and integrate new information and experiences. During our somatic therapy journey, we might experience sometimes intense emotional and physical stuff that requires time for the brain to… well, just rest. Rest can help in forming new neural pathways that support healing and resilience.

2. **Reduction of Stress Hormones**

    Continuous therapeutic activities can sometimes elevate stress hormones, such as cortisol. Rest days provide a break and allow our cortisol levels to normalize. This is, as we well can imagine, vital for preventing burnout and promoting overall mental health.

3. Neuroplasticity

The brain's ability to reorganize itself by forming new neural connections is even boosted with periods of rest. We are often so busy thinking being busy is the key, but many times it's the contrary. Neuroplasticity, as we know, is a critical component of healing from trauma, as it allows the brain to develop new, healthier patterns of thinking and reacting.

Emotional Regulation

Rest days help in regulating emotions by giving the amygdala (the brain's emotional center) time to recover. This regulation is essential in trauma therapy to manage our emotional responses and maintain a balanced state of mind.

4. Enhanced Memory and Learning

Adequate rest improves memory consolidation and learning. In somatic therapy, this means that the therapeutic techniques and coping strategies learned during the healing journey are better retained and applied in daily life.

Overall, incorporating rest days into a somatic therapy program is essential for optimizing the brain's ability to heal from trauma, promoting sustainable recovery, and preventing the negative effects of prolonged stress. Beautiful, right?

So, by just resting, you may sometimes help more than... not resting.

Just ideas for you today:

Where do you see beauty today?

DAY 15: REFLECT ON ANY SHIFTS IN YOUR BODY AWARENESS AND EMOTIONAL STATE

We are halfway, my dear. How does it make you feel?

Again, I wanted to give you a day to just reflect and rest. You are healing, my dear, and your body and mind (and soul, if you ask me) are *healing*.

Today, you can reflect your healing through the lens of your body awareness and emotional state.

Reflect the tools what have helped you so far, the most. Consider how you can take them a beautiful part of your daily life.

If you want, you can gently observe your breathing, or movement, or gentle thoughts today. How do them affect how you feel?

I will give you one question today:

What could bring you joy today?

DAY 16-20: SELF-COMPASSION AND ACCEPTANCE

Ah, now we are talking. Research illuminates how somatic therapies can harness the body's innate wisdom, acknowledging its role as a repository of experiences and emotions.

Studies reveal the transformative power of self-compassion, showing significant reductions in stress, shame, and increased coping self-efficacy. Moreover, acceptance is an incredibly important component in healing, fostering resilience and integration of traumatic experiences.

Somatic therapy can teach us to tune into our body and rely on it as a source of wisdom. So, are you ready to make friends with yourself?

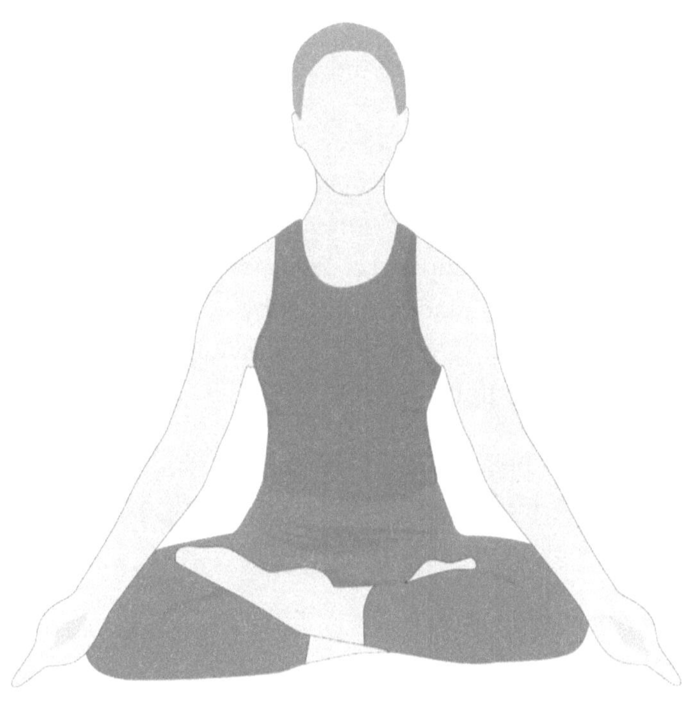

Figure 8 Sit in peace, my dear. If it feels difficult in the beginning, don't worry, with practice you'll be better. Sitting in peace, meditation, breath work, will free up so much space in your... thoughts and feelings.

DAY 16: PRACTICE SELF-COMPASSION MEDITATION, OFFERING KINDNESS TO YOURSELF

Find your place of peace, loving kindness, and acceptance.

Sit comfortably and close your eyes. Observe your breathing, just gently let your consciousness rest in your breathing rhythm. Whenever you are ready, visualize yourself surrounded by a warm, golden light, bathing you in love and compassion. Allow yourself to receive this love fully, knowing that you deserve it simply by being human. Take a few moments to bask in this feeling of unconditional acceptance and kindness toward yourself. [pause]

Take a few deep breaths, and let the unconditional acceptance and kindness really sink in. [pause] When you are ready, you can open your eyes.

How do you feel? Do you notice a difference?

Self-Compassion Letter Writing

Take a few moments to reflect on a difficult experience or emotion you've been struggling with lately. Then, grab a pen and paper and write a letter to yourself **from a place of loving kindness and acceptance**. Acknowledge your pain or suffering with empathy and understanding, validating your emotions without judgment. Remind yourself that imperfection is part of the human experience and that you are worthy of compassion and acceptance, just as you are.

Journaling prompts to help you find your self-compassion and acceptance:

1. Describe a moment when you felt true self-compassion and acceptance towards yourself. What led to this experience?

2. Are there any parts of yourself that you struggle to accept or show kindness towards? Explore why this might be the case.

3. Think about a time when you received compassion from someone else. How did it feel, and how can you offer the same level of compassion to yourself?

4. Consider your self-talk and inner dialogue. Are there any recurring phrases or thoughts that hinder your self-compassion and acceptance?

DAY 17: CULTIVATE GRATITUDE BY FOCUSING ON THE SENSATIONS OF APPRECIATION

My pre-therapy self was unfortunately on constant autopilot, which means I didn't know to pay attention to my triggers and even less to work to heal them.

My post-therapy self and my professional-counselor self knows how important it is not only to do the work, but also to practice gratitude. We have a reason for the saying "count your blessings."

Practicing gratitude is not just some hippie thing; it has real scientifically proven health benefits. Practicing gratitude as part of somatic therapy can offer numerous benefits—and hear this—supported by scientific research:

1. **Neurological Changes**

    Gratitude stimulates the brain's reward system, leading to increased production of dopamine and serotonin, neurotransmitters associated with happiness and wellbeing.

2. **Physical Health**

    Gratitude practice has been linked to lower inflammatory

markers and improved immune function, contributing to overall physical health.

3. **Emotional Regulation**

   Gratitude enhances emotional regulation by fostering positive emotions and reducing stress, anxiety, and depression.

4. **Social Connection**

   Grateful individuals tend to have better social relationships due to their positive outlook and willingness to express appreciation, leading to increased social support and satisfaction.

5. **Spiritual Wellbeing**

   Gratitude is associated with spiritual wellbeing, contributing to better mood, sleep, self-efficacy, and overall psychological health.

Integrating gratitude into your somatic therapy journey can amplify its therapeutic effects by promoting holistic wellbeing, enhancing emotional resilience, and fostering a deeper mind-body connection. Not bad, don't you think?

What moments bring you true joy, and how can you invite them more into your life?

DAY 18: DEEPENING THE SENSATION OF GRATITUDE

Gratitude can be so healing I wanted to dedicate two days for it on this program. Today we practice deepening the feelings of gratitude.

1. **Gratitude Focus**

   Bring to your mind something you're grateful for. It could be a person, an experience, or simply the present moment. Allow yourself to fully immerse in the feeling of gratitude.

2. **Sensory Awareness**

   Pay attention to how gratitude manifests in your body. Notice any physical sensations that arise, such as warmth in your chest, tingling in your fingertips, or a sense of lightness.

3. **Amplification**

   Once you've identified these sensations, amplify them by bringing your full awareness to them. Imagine them expanding and spreading throughout your body.

4. **Integration**

   Take a few moments to integrate this feeling of gratitude into your being. Allow it to infuse every cell of your body, filling you with a profound sense of appreciation.

5. **Reflection**

   After the exercise, take a moment to reflect on how you feel. Notice any shifts in your mood, mindset, or overall sense of wellbeing.

DAY 19: EXPLORE ANY AREAS OF RESISTANCE OR DISCOMFORT WITH GENTLE CURIOSITY

In somatic therapy, exploring areas of resistance and discomfort with gentle curiosity is an important aspect of the healing process.

Why? Because the judgement often comes first, and for our

wellbeing it would be much more beneficial to approach our feelings, even the resistance and discomfort, with loving gentleness. (Or do you know anyone actually benefiting for crucifying themselves constantly?)

By approaching these sensations with openness and non-judgment, we can deepen our understanding of underlying issues and grow self-awareness. This process involves appreciating a mindful awareness of our bodily sensations and exploring them with a sense of curiosity, allowing for integrating emotional experiences. Through these instructions, we can learn to navigate challenging sensations with compassion and self-acceptance, empowering personal growth and healing.

To explore areas of resistance or discomfort with gentle curiosity in somatic therapy, follow these steps:

1. **Awareness**

   Begin by bringing awareness to any sensations of resistance or discomfort in your body. Notice where you feel tension, tightness, or any other physical sensations that signal discomfort.

2. **Curiosity**

   Approach these sensations with gentle curiosity rather than judgment or criticism. Allow yourself to be open to whatever arises without trying to change or fix anything.

3. **Breathwork**

   Use deep, slow breaths to help anchor yourself in the present moment and create a sense of safety. Breathing deeply can also help to release tension and invite a greater sense of relaxation.

4. **Exploration**

With an attitude of curiosity, gently explore the sensations in your body. Notice any thoughts, emotions, or memories that may arise as you focus on the discomfort.

5. **Non-judgment**

Practice non-judgment towards whatever arises during this exploration process. Allow yourself to observe and experience without attaching labels or stories to your sensations.

6. **Validation**

Validate your experience by acknowledging that it is okay to feel discomfort and resistance. Recognize that these sensations are natural responses that serve a purpose in your healing journey.

7. **Integration**

Finally, integrate what you've learned from this exploration into your overall somatic therapy process. Use this newfound awareness to inform your future sessions and deepen your understanding of yourself.

Good work, my dear!

DAY 20: EMBRACE ACCEPTANCE OF YOUR BODY AND EMOTIONS AS THEY ARE NOW

By acknowledging and welcoming our bodily sensations and emotional experiences without judgment, we cultivate a compassionate relationship with ourselves. This process allows for a deeper understanding of the mind-body connection and helps to strengthen our resilience in facing life's challenges. Through somatic techniques such as mindfulness, body scanning, and gentle movement, we can learn to honor our present experiences with a sense of peace and wholeness.

By acknowledging and welcoming our bodily sensations and emotional experiences without judgment, we cultivate a compassionate relationship with ourselves. This process allows for a deeper understanding of the mind-body connection and helps to strengthen our resilience in facing life's challenges. Through somatic techniques such as mindfulness, body scanning, and gentle movement, we can learn to honor our present experiences with a sense of peace and wholeness.

With these instructions you can find your way to welcome your bodily sensations with love and compassion.

1. **Find a Comfortable Space**

   Sit or lie down in a comfortable position where you feel relaxed and safe. Close your eyes if it helps you focus inward.

2. **Connect with Your Breath**

   Like always, begin by taking a few deep breaths, allowing yourself to settle into the present moment. Notice the sensations of your breath as it enters and leaves your body.

3. **Body Scan**

   Slowly scan your body from head to toe, paying attention to any areas of tension, discomfort, or sensation. As you scan, remind yourself that all sensations are valid and part of your experience.

4. **Emotional Check-In**

   Tune into your emotions without judgment. Notice what emotions are present in your body. Allow yourself to feel whatever arises without trying to change it.

5. **Practice Self-Compassion**

Offer yourself kindness and compassion for whatever you're experiencing, both physically and emotionally. Remind yourself that it's okay to feel the way you do.

6. **Affirm Acceptance**

Silently affirm acceptance of your body and emotions as they are at this moment. If you want, you can repeat a simple affirmation such as, "I accept myself exactly as I am right now."

7. **Grounding**

Finally, bring your awareness back to the present moment by feeling the support of the ground beneath you or the surface you're sitting or lying on. Wiggle your toes or gently stretch if it feels good.

8. **Closure**

Take a moment to acknowledge your experience and thank yourself for taking this time for self-care and acceptance.

JOURNALING QUESTIONS TO HELP YOU REFLECT:

1. Imagine your ideal relationship with your body and self. What steps can you take to cultivate this relationship?

2. How can you incorporate gentle self-care practices into your daily routine to nurture gratitude?

DAY 21-25: CONNECTION AND SUPPORT

Day 21-24: Practice Empathetic Communication with Yourself and Others

The reason I wanted you to focus on this for twenty-eight days, is simple. The role of empathetic listening (both ourselves and others) is so incredibly important.

Do you remember or can you imagine how you feel when someone is really listening to you in an empathetic and loving way?

Yes, it's called a deep connection.

Empathetic listening often brings a deep emotional connection, validation, and healing.

It brings validation and safety. Empathetic listening creates a safe space for us and others to express both our and their emotions and experiences without judgment. In somatic therapy, this validation is essential for us to feel heard and understood, promoting trust and openness.

Also, by practicing active listening and empathetic communication with ourselves, we can nurture self-awareness, emotional regulation, and resilience. This internal dialogue fosters a deeper understanding of our personal experiences in a healing way.

DAY 25: REFLECT ON THE ROLE OF SOCIAL CONNECTION IN SUPPORTING SOMATIC HEALING

Social Connections Can Support Somatic Healing

A deep sense of belonging might be the most beautiful and healing thing we can experience in life.

Brené Brown has put it beautifully: *"Owning our story can be hard but not nearly as difficult as spending our lives running from it. Embracing our vulnerabilities is risky but not nearly as dangerous as giving up on love and belonging and joy—the experiences that make us the most vulnerable. Only when we are brave enough to explore the darkness, will we discover the infinite power of our light."*

1. **Emotional Support**

    Social connections are so important! They provide a crucial foundation for somatic healing in a form of emotional support. Sharing experiences and feelings with others creates a sense of understanding and validation, which can ease emotional distress and, of course, support the healing process.

2. **Sense of Belonging**

    Being part of a supportive social network can form a deep sense of belonging and acceptance, which both can be deeply beneficial for somatic healing. Feeling connected to others reduces feelings of isolation and loneliness, promoting psychological wellbeing and resilience during the healing journey. Brene Brown has written beautifully about true, deep belonging, if you want to check her out.

3. **Stress Reduction**

    Social connections can act as buffers against stress, helping somatic healing. Engaging in positive social interactions releases oxytocin and reduces cortisol levels, promoting relaxation and reducing the physiological burden on the body.

4. **Enhanced Coping Mechanisms**

    Strong social connections provide us with coping mechanisms to navigate challenges associated with somatic healing. Supportive relationships offer practical help, advice, and encouragement, empowering us to cope with our physical and emotional struggles.

5. **Promotion of Mind-Body Integration**

Social connections can reinforce our mind-body connection in a beautiful way. Interacting with supportive others can promote self-awareness, mindfulness, and embodiment practices that facilitate healing on both physical and emotional levels.

JOURNALING PROMPTS TO HELP YOU EXPLORE YOUR SOCIAL CONNECTIONS IN YOUR SOMATIC JOURNEY:

1. What role have social connections played in your healing journey, both emotionally and physically?

2. How do you nurture and maintain supportive social connections in your life?

3. Describe a time when you provided support to someone else and how it contributed to both their emotional and physical healing.

4. Reflect on the importance of reciprocal relationships in somatic healing. How do you give and receive support within your social circle?

DAY 26-30: INTEGRATION AND MOVING FORWARD

Now we bring together the insights and experiences you have gained throughout our journey together.

We are in the integration phase of our journey in somatic therapy. Integration in somatic therapy encompasses the harmonization of mind, body, emotions, and behaviors, aiming to bring you profound healing and transformation.

1. **Embracing Wholeness**

Through somatic therapy, you've embarked on this courageous journey of self-discovery, exploring the intricate connection between your physical sensations, emotions, and thoughts. Integration allows you to embrace your wholeness, honoring all aspects of yourself.

2. **Unification of Experiences**

By integrating fragmented experiences, you've cultivated resilience and coherence, paving the way for a more aligned and authentic way of being.

3. **Empowerment:**

As you continue to integrate somatic practices into your daily life, remember the empowerment that comes from embodying your experiences fully. You are equipped with tools to navigate life's challenges with greater ease and presence.

DAY 26: CREATE A SOMATIC SELF-CARE PLAN FOR CONTINUED PRACTICE BEYOND THE PROGRAM

I would really like you to have all the possible healing tools for your days to come. That's why I wanted to stop here for a moment with the integration phase for you to prepare yourself for the future.

If you have a somatic self-care plan, it's so much easier to go on and have a safe feeling of security, even for the challenging days (there will still be those, I'm afraid, for all of us).

You can, for example, use the RAIN technique. It's simple to remember and can help you deeply.

The RAIN technique is a mindfulness practice developed to deal with difficult emotions. Here's how it works:

1. **Recognize**

   Acknowledge the emotion you're experiencing without judgment. Identify what you're feeling.

2. **Allow**

   Accept the presence of the emotion without trying to suppress or ignore it. Allow yourself to feel it fully.

3. **Investigate**

   Explore the emotion with curiosity and kindness. Understand its causes and how it manifests in your body and mind.

4. **Nurture**

   Offer yourself compassion and care. Respond to the emotion with gentleness and self-kindness, soothing yourself as needed.

You might also benefit from a titration technique:

Titration in somatic therapy involves slowing down the process to address trauma renegotiation effectively. Here's a concise overview:

1. **Definition**
   Titration means slowing things down in therapy, addressing trauma's overwhelming nature.

2. **Process**
   It involves determining the pace and amount of work to handle, empowering us and providing a beautiful space for healing.

3. **Benefits**

    Titration enables (trauma) healing by addressing responses in tiny, manageable portions, leaving the rest for later sessions.

DAY 27: ONWARDS: SOME SOMATIC COPING SKILLS, JUST IN CASE

I can't just see you off without giving you some more somatic therapy tools, just in case. If any of the methods in this book resonate with you, you are welcome to take it with you. That's the reason I wrote this book!

Somatic coping skills are more than just techniques; they are tender companions on the road to support your emotional wellbeing. Through these practices — and some extra ones! — and connection, we learn to listen to our bodies, even the whispers, and respond with kindness and understanding.

Every step we take is a step aiming to help your healing. May we embrace ourselves with the same tenderness we would offer to a cherished friend, honoring our journey with patience, grace, and abundant love.

(By the way, just a side note: I was once asked a question when I felt I had messed up something and I was very judgmental towards myself. The question was, "How would you talk to your loved one if they were in your shoes?" Guess how I felt my tone changing. You can try it, too. Talk to yourself like you would to a dear friend.)

The scientific basis of somatic coping skills lies in their efficacy in treating trauma and stress-related disorders. Somatic therapies, such as somatic experiencing (SE), focus on the body's physical sensations to address emotional and psychological trauma. Studies on somatic experiencing are still emerging but show promising results. While more research is needed, existing literature supports the therapeutic value of somatic coping skills in promoting holistic healing and wellbeing.

SENSORY GROUNDING

This helps to bring you to the present moment, even when times are tough. If you feel overwhelmed or stressed, do this:

Name five things you can see, hear, and smell. Name one thing you can touch. How does it feel?

SHAKE IT

Now we shake our worries and stresses off! Begin by finding a comfortable and quiet space where you can move freely. Stand with your feet hip-width apart and take a few deep breaths to center yourself. Then, gently start shaking your arms, allowing the movement to spread throughout your entire body. Embrace any sensations that arise and focus on releasing tension and stress with each shake. Continue shaking for at least three to five minutes, gradually slowing down before coming to a gentle stop. Take a moment to notice compassionately how your body feels afterward.

ANCHOR SAFETY

This safety anchor can go with you everywhere you go. Choose a small object you wear that represents safety for you. It can be a necklace, or a ring, or just a gesture you do with your hands. (I use placing my hand on my heart, I have done it enough times when I meditate, that it instantly calms my heart rate when I do it in a stressful situation, too.)

You can do the same. Literally, you can anchor feelings of safety and joy to your safety anchor. When you feel stressed, focus on your safety object, and let it remind you of your inner strength.

JOURNALING PROMPTS TO HELP YOU EXPLORE SOMATIC COPING SKILLS:

How do you feel about somatic coping skills? Did you try any of them?

Which one of the presented methods invites you the most?

Think about a time when you felt deeply connected to your body and experienced a sense of calm and peace. What activities or practices helped you cultivate this somatic awareness? How can you integrate them into your daily routine?

DAY 28: REVIEW THE SOMATIC EXERCISES THAT RESONATED WITH YOU

Based on your experience with this book, create your very own personalized somatic practice that involves the exercises that resonated with you the most. Develop a routine that fits your lifestyle and commit to integrating somatic practices into your daily or weekly wellness regimen for optimal benefits. Trust me, my dear, you will thank yourself later.

Here is a few more, just in case:

RESOURCING

Resourcing is the somatic practice of inviting our mind/body to attune to the beautiful sensations of safety or goodness, no matter how small they may be. The process of attending to a felt sense of "okayness" begins teaching our nervous system that stress is ok, and from the stress we can then come back to calmness. (My dear, it is possible.) Especially if you experience high stress, it is helpful to have a plan to connect back to the peace and calmness.

(And… self-hug. See the next page.

Yes, you read it right, my dear! Self-hugging can be incredible healing. As mammals, we need touching, and if no-one is around, we can help ourselves to calm our nervous system with self-hug, for example. There is actual science backing this up.)

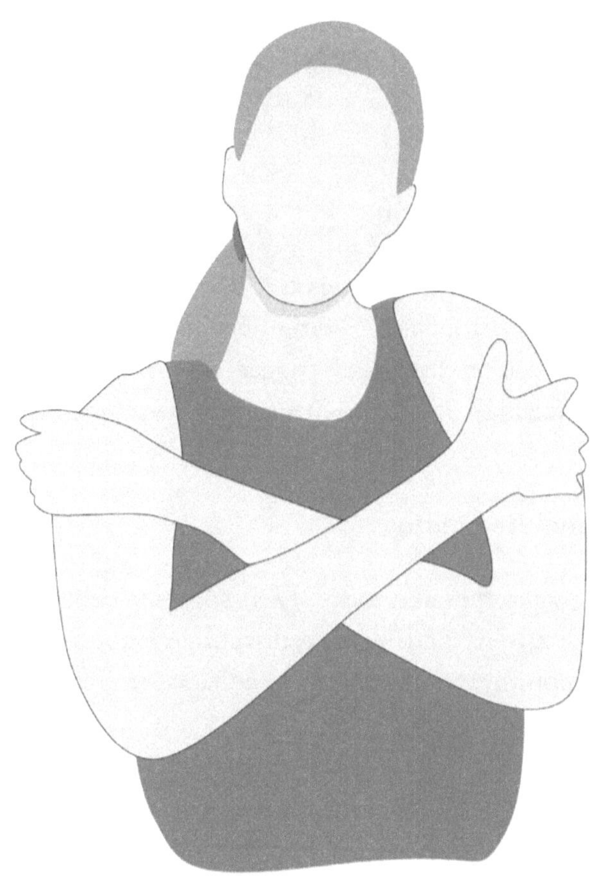

Figure 9: Yes, you read it right. Self-hugging can be incredible healing!

SELF-HUG

THE SCIENCE OF SELF-HUGGING IN SOMATIC THERAPY

1. **Cortisol Reduction**

   Research indicates that self-soothing touch, including self-hugging, can lead to a reduction in our cortisol levels. Cortisol, of course, is a stress hormone. This suggests that engaging in self-hugging can help regulate the body's stress response and find a sense of calmness.

2. **Activation of Oxytocin**

   Oxytocin, often referred to as the "love hormone," is released during physical touch, including hugging. Studies have shown that self-hugging can also trigger the release of oxytocin, bringing feelings of security, trust, and relaxation with it. Not bad?

3. **Emotional Regulation**

   Self-hugging serves as a form of self-soothing behavior, helping us reduce anxiety and regulate disruptive emotions. Providing physical comfort to ourselves can enhance emotional resilience and overall wellbeing.

4. **Somatic Experiencing**

   While the specific scientific research on self-hugging within somatic therapy is limited, somatic experiencing techniques often incorporate self-soothing practices like self-hugging to help us regulate their nervous system and process traumatic experiences. These techniques aim to restore a sense of safety and connection within the body, and to heal trauma.

Self-hugging, as a somatic therapy tool, combines both physiological and psychological mechanisms to bring relaxation, emotional regulation, and stress reduction, ultimately supporting our holistic wellbeing.

Consider journaling your thoughts on this:

What practises and exercises did you feel most comfortable with?

Why do you think they were the ones you liked the most?

How do you think they can help you the most?

EXTRA DAY 29: SET INTENTIONS FOR YOUR SOMATIC AWARENESS FROM NOW ON

Intention, again, is the magic word. You can reflect on how you see your future healing with your deepened somatic awareness, and how you will continue healing with it.

AGAIN, CONSIDER JOURNALING YOUR THOUGHTS ON THIS:

Reflect on your personal experiences with somatic exercises. Consider any past experiences in which you've had difficult moments and compare them to more recent ones. Do you feel you have changed on your courageous somatic journey? Identify the techniques that have helped you the most to manage stress, improve relaxation, or enhance your mind-body connection, and continue this path, my dear! You are a super star.

EXTRA DAY 30: CELEBRATE YOUR JOURNEY AND GROWTH (WE CELEBRATE WITH YOU!)

You are a superhero, my dear. You did it, the whole journey what we had for you in this book. How do you feel, today?

I deeply hope this book has brought you the peace and love you deserve. I hope it has helped to guide you in deeper connection with your mind and body, and you have found a sparkling, loving presence in your body. May you carry with you the profound understanding that you have the inner knowing.

Remember, you had the courage to seek healing. As you embark on the next chapter of your journey, may you continue to honor the wisdom of your body, listen to its whispers, and trust in its innate ability to heal. May you find comfort in knowing that you have the strength and resilience to overcome adversity and emerge stronger and more alive than ever before.

With deep gratitude for accompanying us on this transformative voyage, we wish you well, hoping that the seeds of healing will continue to flourish and bloom in your soul.

(And I deeply hope we meet again. There will be more books.)

PART IV

"No one is you and that is your Superpower".
—Unknown

Our 28-day experience (with few extras) is about to end.

How do you feel today, my dear?

I hope you are proud of yourself. **I am soooooooo proud of you!**

Remember Karen, who had been bullied at work when she was in her twenties? I guided her to this program, and it helped her release a lot of tension and stored trauma from her body. When her body was liberated from the unconscious trauma, her mind got liberated too.

She began to flourish! Her eyes sparkled, and she transformed, literally in front of my eyes.

Of course, healing from traumas takes time. It's a process with ups and downs, and with courage and love, we can heal from traumas, too.

POST-JOURNEY SELF-ASSESSMENT

As we promised, we will give you an opportunity to explore your journey as a self-assessment. The questions are identical for a purpose: answering the same questions before and after your journey may help you to compare the answers before and after and see how much you have changed.

This may provide insights into the overall effectiveness of our journey together and the extent of healing that you feel has occurred.

1. On a scale of 1-10, how would you rate your overall level of physical tension or discomfort?

2. How intense are your bodily sensations when experiencing stress or anxiety? Rate from 1 to 10.

3. To what extent do you feel connected to your body on a daily basis? Rate from 1 (not at all) to 10 (very connected).

4. How would you rate your awareness of bodily sensations, such as muscle tension or heart rate changes? Use a scale of 1-10.

5. On a scale of 1-10, how present are you in your body during moments of emotional distress?

6. How comfortable do you feel expressing emotions physically (e.g., through gestures or body movements)? Rate from 1 to 10.

7. To what extent do you notice changes in your breathing patterns during times of stress? Rate from 1 (not noticeable) to 10 (highly noticeable).

8. How frequently do you experience physical symptoms, such as headaches or stomachaches, related to stress or emotional triggers? Rate from 1 to 10.

9. On a scale of 1-10, how often do you notice feelings of joy and peace?

10. To what extent do you feel grounded and present in your body? Use a scale of 1-10.

ANALYSIS AND INTERPRETATION

See the answers you gave in the initial and post-therapy assessments. The scores you have may identify trends and improvements. Some areas may still require attention, and with these assessments, you will have an idea what those can be.

DOCUMENTATION AND FOLLOW-UP

Document the findings of the self-assessment evaluations and any relevant observations. You may, if you feel you want, continue monitoring your progress even after this journey. You can do these questions regularly, if you wish.

CONCLUSION

"Your body listens to everything your mind says. Be kind to yourself."

— Unknown

I hope, if nothing else, this book has helped guide you to embrace deep love towards yourself. *You deserve it.*

If we all had the courage you have, the world would be a better place.

If we all leaned towards the difficult and took the journey in the unknown, we would have so much love on the planet.

I hope you feel how proud I am of you!

I hope you feel proud of yourself.

I hope you found the scientific facts about somatic therapy come to life in your experience, supporting and guiding you into deep healing.

You might want to continue your healing journey, and if you do, I hope you know I will always be there for you. My passion is to help others. I consider it my life calling, and I feel deep gratitude when someone can benefit from my work.

Wherever you decide to go next, please be kind to yourself. Honor your boundaries and safe space, and trust your inner guidance.

I could write a whole book about the inner wisdom that lives inside of us all, if we take the time to listen.

You listened to your guidance and took a brave step to heal. Thank you for choosing us, from all the thousands and thousands of alternatives.

I hope you found what your guidance led you to explore. I hope you found a spark of empowerment, which can have room to grow inside you.

I would like to leave you with these beautiful words that some wise unknown beautiful person said: *Those who believe in magic, tend to find it.*

I hope you have found and will find your magic.

It does exist.

It exists in beautiful sunrises, in a child's laughter, it shows itself in a raindrop, or the first beautiful cup of coffee in the morning (my first coffee tends to be magical, and I always try to take a moment and really taste it). The magic lies in the simple things of life. It's in the forests, or beach, or a selfless smile of a stranger.

I remember once when we were driving in France and our car broke down. (A side note: if you want adventure, go on a ten-thousand-mile road trip—yes, it's ten thousand miles, you read it right—in an old car, with two small kids and not too much money with you.) Standing by the road in the French Alps, within five minutes we had a stranger pulling over and guiding us to the repair shop, making sure we understood everything they told us. The wife of the repair guy brought our kids old toys that their children had been playing with a decade or two or three ago. They made sure we had something to eat. (OMG, French pastries are gorgeous!) They did everything they possibly could to help us, even when we didn't speak French. (If I had a bucket list, learning to speak French would be on it.)

There is so much beautiful magic, all around us.

When we slowly heal, we can see it better.

In the French car shop, I had to consciously remind myself to get out of my initial reflex that the world is a dangerous place. I managed to breathe myself calm, even when it felt difficult, and it turned out to be a beautiful experience. I hope this book helped you on your journey to the beauty.

I hope this book helped you to feel the care I have for you.

I hope you have found ways to regulate your nervous system to feel the beauty of life.

You are a rock star.

I wanted to share this for you to understand where I came from. I had a difficult childhood with toxic and abusive parents. I grew up thinking when I leave this house, I want to help others so that no-one has to experience what I did. I studied psychology from early on, as well as somatic methods, because I felt they helped me.

Like Rumi so beautifully said: *The wound is where the Light enters.*

Trauma healing is a process.

I do believe we all meet at the right time, with the right people, or books, or movies, if you will. I believe we are guided. It gives me comfort to think there is a higher power who looks after us. (The higher power does sometimes have a very particular sense of humor, though, but that's a topic to another book.)

I have listened to a lot of spiritual and scientific leaders and followed their work—and especially spiritual leaders with a scientific touch, and scientific leaders with a spiritual touch. They all say in one form or another: *our pasts lead us to this moment.*

I have heard about people who get a mystical experience, and they can see their lives in a bigger context, and they all say afterwards, they firstly fall in love with the person (which is themselves), and they can clearly see all the pain points leading their lives to that point. And they praise all those moments of pain and difficulty and sadness. Because they know, it was those moments that led them to this moment. It wasn't all the happy happy joy joy moments of their lives; it was the difficult ones.

If we looked at life, even from the theoretical point of view, what if we learned to understand all our lives and all of life's experiences lead us to this moment, would it give us comfort? Would it give us a feeling of safety? Love?

But wait, I Want You to Have Some Bonus Material

And finally, as our journey together in this book comes towards the final pages (but not the end, I hope!), I wanted to give you some extras, just in case. (I know, I sound like a mom who's child is moving away from home, and I kind of feel like that, wanting to make sure you are ok. And remember, I am here if you need anything, I will write to you more!)

Here you can find the longer body scan meditation script as I promised earlier.

BONUS 1: BODY SCAN MEDITATION (A LONGER VERSION)

Let's begin by finding a comfortable position. You can sit in a chair, ensuring your back is straight yet relaxed, with your feet planted firmly on the ground. Alternatively, you may choose to stand or lie down with your head supported. Allow your hands to rest gently in your lap or by your side. Close your eyes softly, or maintain a relaxed gaze.

[pause]

Now, let's take a few slow, deep breaths, inhaling through your nose and exhaling through your nose or mouth. Feel your abdomen expand with each inhale and relax as you exhale. Gradually shift your focus from external distractions to your inner self, gently tuning in to your breath.

[pause]

Direct your attention to your feet, noticing any sensations present. You might wiggle your toes, feeling the subtle movements against your socks or shoes. Imagine your breath flowing down to your feet, nurturing them with each inhale and releasing tension with each exhale.

[pause]

As you feel ready, let your awareness travel upward to your ankles, calves, knees, and thighs, observing the sensations throughout your legs. With each breath, breathe into and out of your legs, acknowledging any discomfort without judgment.

[pause]

Continue this mindful exploration, moving up through your lower back, pelvis, mid-back, and upper back. Notice any sensations in your muscles, temperature variations, or points of contact with your surroundings. With each exhale, release any tension you may be holding.

[pause]

Shift your focus to your abdomen, noticing the sensations within. Become aware of your chest and heart region, observing the rhythm of your heartbeat. Then, bring your attention to your hands and fingertips, breathing into and out of this area.

[pause]

Transition your awareness to your arms, neck, shoulders, and throat, allowing any tension to soften and dissolve with each exhale. Finally, notice the sensations in your scalp, head, and face, releasing any remaining tension.

[pause]

Expand your awareness to encompass your entire body from head to toe, feeling the gentle flow of your breath throughout. Take a deep breath, drawing in the energy of your practice, and exhale fully.

[pause]

When you feel ready, gently open your eyes and return to the present moment. Consider setting an intention for this practice to benefit not only yourself but also those around you.

BONUS 2: 10 SIMPLE WAYS TO IMPROVE YOUR HEALTH

I wanted to give you my dear mom's wise words. Unfortunately, she is not here with us anymore (Oh, how I miss her!), but I hope her words will support and guide also you.

When I still was living with my parents, my mom used to always ask me two questions, no matter what situation I was in. They were, "Have you remembered to eat?" And the other, "Have you slept?"

When my husband and I lost our child, in my heart, I heard my mom asking those exact questions. Have you remembered to eat? Have you slept?

The answer, of course, was "no" to both of the questions, and the more I had stress, the more it was a "no." Now I know how unbelievably important it is. The more the boat rocks, the more important it is to take care of those basic things.

I wanted to offer you 10 simple ways you can easily improve your health, and now the science backs up my mom's questions: The simple things are often the most important. From my point of view, pretty much all the health experts have similar types of lists, including Harvard Health, and other professionals. There might be some minor variations, and the order might vary, but here are the basics. Please consider making a habit out of them, and I can promise you'll feel so much better.

1. **Breathe.**

    Breathing is a tool we carry around at all times. Learn breathing techniques and find the ones best suited for you. You can find breathing technique instructions in this book. Please consider doing them!

2. **Strech in the mornings.**

It will set your body for the day, wake it up gently, and improve your circulation, as well as promote relaxation. For gentle stretches you can find instructions in this book, and with the bonuses as part of the 30-Day Somatic Yoga Experience.

3. **Have good sleep, and take naps.**

The power of sleep from the scientific point of view is clear. If you have sleeping problems, consider toning down towards the evening, keep a steady daily rhythm, put away the screens hours before bedtime. And, my dear, take naps! A study published online in Jan. 2021, by General Psychiatry suggests that nappers score higher on cognitive tests than non-nappers.

4. **Shake it a bit!**

Regular physical activity offers numerous health benefits, supported by scientific evidence. Studies show that exercise can reduce the risk of chronic diseases such as cardiovascular disease, cancer, and type 2 diabetes. Physical activity also enhances brain health, aids in weight management, strengthens bones and muscles, and boosts overall wellbeing. Additionally, daily movement not only improves physical health but also has a positive impact on mental wellbeing, contributing to a balanced and healthier lifestyle.

5. **Learn something new.**

The story claims Einstein has once said, "The mind is like a parachute. It only works if it's open." Keep your mind open, my dear. It's not just beneficial for life's quality perspective, but also health-wise.

6. **Stay hydrated.**

Drink plenty of water throughout the day to support bodily functions and maintain hydration.

7. **Nurture loving social connections.**

Foster loving relationships with friends, family, and community to promote mental and emotional wellbeing.

8. **Balance your diet.**

Remember, food is a beautiful, nourishing thing. (You might consider not listening the millions of diet programs with insane requirements.) Include a variety of fruits, vegetables, whole grains, lean proteins, and healthy fats in your meals. Colorful food usually equals healthy food.

9. **Practice stress management.**

Incorporate somatic coping skills or other types of relaxation techniques such as deep breathing, meditation, or yoga to reduce stress levels. There's a saying that goes pretty much like this: meditate 20 minutes every day, unless you are busy, then meditate an hour a day. The idea behind it? Yep, it's doing things from a place of peace.

10. **Practice gratitude.**

The science behind this one is enormous. Remember how gratitude feels in your body. You can close your eyes and feel it. List five things each morning that you are grateful for. It takes five minutes and can change your life. Neuroscientific research indicates that individuals who regularly express gratitude experience enhanced physical health outcomes, such as strengthened immune function and reduced risk of diseases. Furthermore, gratitude practices can lead to structural changes in the brain associated with increased happiness and overall life satisfaction. When we consciously express gratitude, specific neural circuits associated with positive emotions, such as the ventromedial prefrontal cortex (VMPFC) and the anterior cingulate cortex, are activated. This activation triggers the release of neurotransmitters like dopamine, which contribute to feelings of happiness and wellbeing. Regular expressions of gratitude strengthen neural pathways associated with positive emotions and wellbeing. Over time, this rewiring effect can lead to lasting changes in the brain: resilience, emotional balance, and a more optimistic outlook on life. Additionally, gratitude meditation has been shown to induce decreased activation in brain regions associated with stress and anxiety, such as the amygdala, contributing to improved emotional regulation and mental health.

11. Take good care of your teeth.

The benefits of maintaining good dental health go a million miles beyond just your mouth. Actually, oral health has been found as one of the 10 leading health indicators along with other indicators such as nutrition, cancer, HIV, and heart disease for overall access to health.

Please promise me you'll take good care of yourself.

And remember to ask yourself, especially if you are in acute stress: Have I remembered to eat? Have I slept?

Often, when things get complicated and difficult, the simplest things can help the most.

FIND YOUR LOVING SUPPORT GROUP

"When you hear the knock, consider the invitation."
—Lisa Miller, professor, researcher and clinical psychologist and
scientist

I would love to leave you with something beautiful for your mind. I love this meditation from Lisa Miller, a beautiful professor and clinical psychologist who has studied depression and spirituality in our neurology. She honors her teacher, Dr. Gary Weaver, who she says she got it from. (By the way, I love Lisa Miller's work, and I warmly recommend it to anyone.)

I invite you to consider recording this; for example, on your mobile, so it's in your reach every time when you need loving support.

GUIDED MEDITATION: YOUR TABLE

"I want to invite you to close your eyes and clear out your inner space. Take five breaths. I invite you to set before you, the inner chamber in you, a table. To this table you may invite anyone, living or deceased, who truly has your best interest in mind.

[pause]

"Anyone living or deceased, who truly has your best interest in mind. [pause] And with them all sitting there, ask them if they love you.

[pause]

"And now, you may invite your higher self, the part of you that is so much more than anything you have done or not done, anything you have or do not have—your true eternal higher self. [pause] And ask you, if you love you.

[pause]

"And now, finally, you may invite your higher power, however you know, whatever word you may use, you higher power. Ask your higher power, if they love you.

[pause]

"And now, with all of these people sitting there, right now, what do they need to share, what do they need to tell you now—what do you need to know?

[long pause]

"And when you are ready, I invite you to come back.

"Welcome back. Let yourself come to the present moment in peace, just gently observe how do you feel. This is your birth right," says Lisa Miller.

I love every word she says. She says it might vary who shows up to our table, depending on where we are on our journey, and you may ask what is in your heart. She continues that all traditions through time have held an understanding of transcendent relationship with our higher power, our higher self, and those who truly have our best interest in mind.

PART V

REFERENCES

Brown, B (2010). *The Gifts of Imperfection.* Hazelden Publishing.

Divine, M (2016, May 4). *The Breathing Technique a Navy SEAL Uses to Stay Calm and Focused.* Time Magazine. https://time.com/4316151/breathing-technique-navy-seal-calm-focused/

Eagleman, D (2020). *Livewired—the Inside Story of the Ever-Changing Brain.* Canongate Books.

Kolk van der, B (2014). *The Body Keeps The Score. Mind, brain and body in the transformation of trauma.* Penguin Random House.

Levine, P. A (1997). *Waking The Tiger. Healing Trauma.* North Atlantic Books Berkeley, California.

Mate, G (2019). *When The Body Says No. The Cost of Hidden Stress.* Penguin Random House UK.

McKeown, P (2021). *The Breathing Cure.* OxyAt Books.

Miller, L (2021). *The Awakened Brain.* Penguin House.

Nestor, J (2020). Breath. *The New Science of a Lost Art.* Penguin Random House.

Salomon, M (2023, July 7). *What is somatic therapy?* Harvard Health Publishing. https://www.health.harvard.edu/blog/what-is-somatic-therapy-202307072951

Silva, L (2024, February 20). *What Is Somatic Therapy? Benefits, Types And Efficacy.* Forbes. https://www.forbes.com/health/mind/somatic-therapy/

Walter, C. H (2019). *Comparison of surf and hike therapy for active-duty service members with major depressive disorder: Study protocol for a randomized controlled trial of novel interventions in a naturalistic setting.* Contemporary Clinical Trials Communication, Volume 16. https://www.sciencedirect.com/science/article/pii/S2451865419301978

What is TRE. https://traumaprevention.com/what-is-tre/

N. N. (2018, May 13). *How Stress Affects The Body.* HeartMath Institute. https://www.heartmath.com/blog/health-and-wellness/how-stress-affects-the-body/

PODCASTS

(2020, July 20). Change Your Brain: Neuroscientist Dr. Andrew Huberman. RichRoll. https://www.youtube.com/watch?v=SwQhKFMxmDY&t=2s

Shetty, J (2023 May 29). *Dr. Joe Dispenza ON: How To Brainwash Yourself For Success And Destroy Negative Thoughts.* Jay Shetty Podcast. Youtube-video. https://www.youtube.com/watch?v=d7sUWwHugg8

ACKNOWLEDGEMENTS

This book wouldn't have been written without all the beautiful people out there who gave permission for their stories for the goal of helping others. I have, for respect to their privacy, altered their stories a bit, with the main goal of being able to describe their situation for the reader to understand better. I want to express my deepest heartfelt gratitude to you all. Each and every one of you have taught me something and guided me on my path. Thank you.

I am also deeply grateful for those beautiful human beings who have harnessed their intent to help and their sparkling minds to serve. Thank you, all you researchers, authors, professors, and other professionals who have not only passed your professionalism, onwards to others but also inspired, and given strength and courage, among others, for me in my work. I especially want to express my gratitude to some scientific and spiritual leaders who have—in my opinion—boldly followed their hearts to, once again, serve others. Now, I want to underline, these names are not in the order of importance or significance: Brené Brown, Joe Dispenza, Andrew Huberman, Lisa Miller, James Nestor, **Dr. Tara Swart, Dr. Daniel Siegel, Dr. Deepak Chopra, Dr. Ellen Langer, Dr. James Doty and so many others**. The list could go on for hundred pages. Thank you. You have inspired so many people.

We all have a gift to take part in serving others. After all, we all share the experience of this beautiful hike called life, inside our funny little leather bags. Life is so much more meaningful when we have the courage to reach out and connect with ourselves and others.

I am deeply grateful to *you*, my dear. Without *you*, my work as an author would be meaningless. I am deeply touched if this book helped you on your path. That is where I feel my purpose is.

Thank you for giving me an opportunity.

FROM YOUR PUBLISHER

"There are only two places you need to go:
the place that heals you, and the place that inspires you."

–Unknown

We in My Zen Power Tribe Publishing believe in these words. We wanted to create books that both heal and inspire. But we wanted to do more than that. We wanted to create a supportive tribe.

We are women authors, screenwriters and designers. We are psychologists, theologists, screenwriters, and artistic directors—we are moms, coffee enthusiasts, travelers. We take our kids to school; we give big presentations; we are willing to work to keep our minds open. We are imperfect. We look after each other. We are fun and we kick ass.

We have our master's degrees and awards and short listings. Several of our books have hit the Top New Release #1 and/or Best Seller in Amazon right when launched—but mostly we want to see ourselves just simply storytellers and someone right by your side. There is so much magic in life, and we all deserve to experience it. We all share this existence on this planet, inside our funny little leather bags—why not find the beauty of it, together?

If you feel this is for you, welcome, my dear. We have a mission: to turn humankind into kind humans—one smile, one healed heart, one sense of true belonging at a time.

You deserve love and joy, my dear. Welcome.

Remember:
"A glowing woman can help other women glow and still be lit."

— Unknown

With love,

My Zen Power Tribe Publishing crew

FURTHER READING FROM THE PUBLISHER

We believe healing and creating dreams are actually two sides of the same thing, even when they may sometimes seem they are not.

Let me tell you why.

From our perspective, healing can lead to a dream life, and creating a dream life can lead to healing. A clear situation of a total **win-win**!

We want you to have all the chances to get what you most want in life, and that's why we have created books for both healing and creating dreams into reality.

Healing

Trauma Work Series
Somatic Therapy Work Series
Shadow Work Guidebook Series (also large print version)

Creating Your Dream Life

Vision Board Book Series for Women

Welcome to explore a continuation for your beautiful journey at amazon.com/author/my_zen_power_tribe

Your Free Gift: A Step-By-Step Guide to Create Your Dream Life

We wanted to remind you of your **free** gift, if you didn't claim it yet.

We do believe healing and creating our dream life is actually very close to one another, since dreams (or goals, if you will) can fuel our healing and vice versa. Sometimes looking to the future is as important as looking and healing from our past.

We want to give you tools to help you create your dream life.

You can have the tools by signing in our website www.myzenpower.co

And you will get a FREE eBook, a Step-By-Step Guide To Create Your Dream Life!

But there is more! You will also get sneak peaks, free copies of our future books, healing information... plus a loving tribe of like-minded friends on the same journey. Welcome, my dear.

We hope this journey we share is only the first journey together. We believe in creating our dream lives, and it can happen through healing and, for example, envisioning our dream life—we believe we all are worth finding the magic in our lives.

Thank You!

Once again, thank you for this journey. I hope you feel how proud I am of you.